Praise for *Reboot Your Brain*

'At a time when research on the development of traditional pharmaceutical treatments for dementia are being abandoned, 'Reboot Your Brain' offers an exhilarating and deep look into the lifestyle and environmental changes that anyone faced with declining brain function can adopt.

Sara Davenport is a brilliant writer and futurist. She offers hope in a compelling and indeed practical and very moving way to all humanity.'

DIPNARINE MAHARAJ MB CHB (GLASG.), MD (GLASG.), FRCP (GLASG.), FRCP (EDIN.), FRCPATH, FACP, MEDICAL DIRECTOR, DBA MAHARAJ INSTITUTE OF IMMUNE REGENERATIVE MEDICINE, USA

'HEALTHY WARNING: reading this book will cause you to make surprising changes to your life without making tough conscious choice. It just gets to you.

Sara has clearly been digging around in the research and data, I just didn't expect her to get inside my data processor, change it a little, and set me off with some new habits and behaviours. It's a really compelling read.'

ADAM TURNER, CHIEF SEE MORE IN OTHERS OFFICER, STANDARD CHARTERED BANK

'Sara has managed to combine accurate and accessible insights from multiple science disciplines with practical tools to provide a reader with both a good understanding of the functioning of the human brain (and how it is connected to other systems) and the steps to take to help it function optimally. Fascinating and very helpful!'

GABIJA TOLEIKYTE, PHD, NEUROSCIENCE, UNIVERSITY COLLEGE, LONDON

'Reboot your Brain offers us an evidenced-based case for making a behavioural change to our lives: diet, exercise and lifestyle... This is the book which can help you make the step change to a new you.'

PROF JONATHAN PASSMORE, PROFESSOR OF COACHING AND BEHAVIOURAL CHANGE, HENLEY BUSINESS SCHOOL, UK

REBOOT
your
Brain

REBOOT
your
Brain

AFRAID OF LOSING YOUR MIND?
UNDERSTAND IT • HEAL IT • FUTURE-PROOF IT

SARA DAVENPORT

REBOOT
PRESS

First published in Great Britain in 2020 by Sara Davenport

Copyright © Sara Davenport 2020

A Cataloguing in Publication record for this book is available from the British Library

Printed by Orphans Press, Leominster

ISBN: 978-1-5272-4626-3

For my father, David
With my love

'It becomes clearer and clearer that we human beings
are not in fact, as we have thought for the past 120
years, psychological systems, but energy systems
instead. And it is energy, in the form of light, sound,
vibration and electricity that our brains respond to.'

SARA DAVENPORT

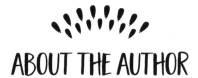

ABOUT THE AUTHOR

S ara Davenport has been at the centre of the wellbeing sector for three decades. In 1998, she set up the charity, Breast Cancer Haven, which is now one of the UK's leading national breast cancer charities with seven centres across the country.

Through her work with doctors, nutritionists and therapists, Sara has an unrivalled view of both traditional and complementary medicine. Her aim is to widen the understanding of how non-invasive, natural approaches to healing can work hand in hand with conventional medical treatments. Her goal is to help each one of us to learn about the fundamental basics of good health, providing inexpensive and effective tools to help you take responsibility for your own wellbeing and live a healthy, happy life.

Sara is the author of *Reboot Your Health: Simple tests and solutions to assess and improve your health (Hay House 2018)*, a holistic DIY manual that helps you establish how well your body is functioning and build a clear and detailed map of what's working and what is not.

She also writes the weekly blog www.reboothealth.co.uk, featuring articles covering an extensive range of health issues and offering simple, but effective, natural solutions.

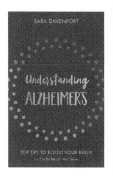
Other Titles...

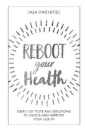  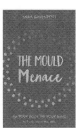 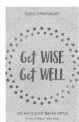 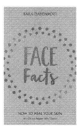

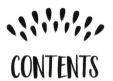

CONTENTS

*'Every man can, if he so desires,
become the sculptor of his own brain.'*

SANTIAGO RAMON Y CAJAL

STEP ONE: UNBURDEN YOUR BRAIN

STEP TWO: REPAIR YOUR BRAIN

STEP THREE: BOOST YOUR BRAIN

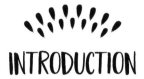

INTRODUCTION

'The root of all health is in the brain. The trunk of it is in emotion. The branches and leaves are the body. The flower of health blooms when all parts work together.'

TRADITIONAL KURDISH SAYING

Brain health has never seemed such a priority. We are facing a tsunami of mental health problems – statistics show that one in four people (in the UK) will suffer from anxiety and depression in any given year. On top of that the dementia epidemic facing our increasingly ageing population has become as frightening as the threat of cancer.

But finding help amongst the range of treatments and preventative options available can be overwhelming – whether you want to reduce damage to your brain or simply protect it against decline. And when you do start to research, it can also seem impossible to keep up with new developments. Every few weeks a new study adds another, often contradictory, 'risk factor' or 'preventative measure' into the mix. So much so that many people feel tempted to simply carry on regardless and ignore all the conflicting advice. But to do so is to let passive avoidance and unhealthy habits rule your life. Why not take a more proactive stance?

I am a fervent believer in the brain–body connection

The brain and its link to all aspects of health has always fascinated me. Breast Cancer Haven, the charity I set up in 1998, has successfully helped many thousands, using a mixture of complementary treatments, talking therapies and nutritional advice. I have spent countless hours talking to our visitors, listening to their stories, and sharing in their concerns. And one important common factor became apparent within weeks of opening the doors of our first centre in London – that many of the patients had experienced a major psychological trauma or shock shortly before their diagnosis. This stoked my curiosity, and I found myself wondering whether there was a more complex relationship between breast cancer, this most physical of illnesses, and what was going on inside the brains of its sufferers.

What is more, the deeper I looked into the benefits of taking a holistic approach to the treatment of cancer that factored in patients' minds as well as bodies and, crucially, acknowledged the impact of stress on both, the stronger my hunch grew. Anecdotally, it was clear from the feedback to the Haven team that our interventions, most of which were focused on the mind-body connection, made a difference to patients at a deep level.

There is now persuasive evidence to back up the benefit of such interventions. One study, whose findings were published in 2018, looked at a group of women suffering from breast cancer, in which half of them were offered group counselling sessions. The results showed that not only was the survival rate in the therapy group significantly higher than in the control group, but recurrence rates were also lower. Similar results have been observed in research relating to the effects of meditation, nutritional interventions and complementary, or alternative, therapies from acupuncture to aromatherapy. I anticipate that future studies, helped by the availability of brain scans, will reveal yet more about the complex inter-relationship between brain, body and disease.

Emerging research

I am interested in anything related to the impact of ageing on the brain and the alternative ways that this process can be slowed or reversed. Since the millennium, scientists have made huge leaps in their understanding of the brain. This explosion of neuroscience research, and the introduction of advanced imaging systems (see pages 217-18), has enabled us to actually see, for the first time, the physically transformative impact that therapeutic and health-boosting activities have had on the brain itself. The brains of those who meditate, exercise, engage in talking therapy, and eat healthily, actually look different to the brains of those who don't. Cynics who had previously dismissed meditation and counselling as 'fluffy' and unscientific, often ascribing any benefits to 'the placebo effect', have been forced to revise their opinions. Meditation training has been widely adopted by schools, some doctors' surgeries, and even some parts of the military. And the impact of nutrition on disease prevention now has a groundswell of solid science behind it.

My greater urgency to look at the options

In tandem with this new credibility for alternative ways to boost physical and mental health, I began to notice more and more headlines about dementia. Dementia is not a specific disease, but a general term used to describe a collection of symptoms that cause a decline in mental ability severe enough to interfere with daily life, of which Alzheimer's disease is the most common. The picture here seemed far bleaker. Older friends and people of my parents' generation began to share news of symptoms and diagnoses. Barely a month went by without word of another family being touched by it. Then, a year ago, my own father was diagnosed with early stages of Alzheimer's. Although he was otherwise fit and well, I had suspected for some time that his memory slips and occasional forgetfulness were a more serious concern than the brain fog that often comes with age.

At first, it felt hopeless – acceptance seems like the only appropriate reaction. There's no cure for Alzheimer's – at best experts predict it is likely to be many decades off – so it's difficult not to receive the news of a diagnosis with sadness and resignation. However, I wasn't prepared to give in entirely, so I resolved to support my father by doing what I do best: to meet the challenge by researching and exploring what was going on outside of conventional medicine.

My father's brain had always been clear as a bell, and despite being in his early 80s, people often remarked on his youthfulness. But, he had begun to lose track of what he was saying mid-sentence, or head off to do something and then retrace his steps a few minutes later, having forgotten what the original task was. He also began to forget the names of people he had known for years. The confusion only lasted for a few minutes, but it was enough to worry him considerably. Then the dread of what might be happening to his mind began to overwhelm him, probably adding considerably to his confusion.

When the doctor gave him the diagnosis, he didn't really seem to take it in. And in view of the fact that there is currently no medical cure, we didn't see the point of adding to his distress by explaining that to him. I know from my years of working with people with cancer, that it's often the shock of the diagnosis and the all-encompassing fear that the diagnosis triggers which overwhelm the person almost more than the disease itself.

There has to be hope

Medical history is full of examples of diseases once deemed incurable, from smallpox to diphtheria, which have been finally conquered by science and are now either manageable or entirely eradicated. The work of the Australian doctor Barry Marshall springs to mind. His claim to have established a bacterial cause of peptic ulcers and gastric cancer was rubbished when it was first suggested in the 1980s. Fast forward to 2005 and he was awarded the Nobel Prize for his research.

So, I know it is merely a question of timing – but will the Alzheimer's cure, the 'holy grail' longed for by sufferers and their families, arrive in time for my father? The odds are against it. Having said that, the exciting work in the USA by Dr Michael Fossel seems like offering a serious possibility. Dr Fossel and his team are working on telomerase gene therapy. Specifically, they are looking at extending the length of your telomeres – the caps at the end of each strand of DNA that protect your chromosomes, like the plastic tips at the end of shoelaces – with a single injection, thereby rejuvenating the age of the brain. They have had consistent success in tests with animal models, showing that aged animals with poor memory, poor learning ability and other poor behavioural measures, have consistently improved in all areas. At the time of writing they are waiting for US Food and Drug Administration (FDA) approval for human trials and searching for funding.[1]

There are also exciting developments in the field of immunology. Tests can now analyse the strengths and weaknesses of your immune system, and highlight precisely which genes are working less than optimally, then tailor treatment to repair any damage. Boost this treatment with stem cells (see reference section, page 273) and the indications are that once your immune system is optimised, diseases, including brain deficiencies, disappear.

What can be done in the meantime?

The best option for both those who already have a dementia diagnosis, and anyone looking toward the future, who simply wants to minimise mental deterioration whatever their age and state of health, has to be to seek out interventions that already exist. Many of these have been developed by small companies with limited funds, and lots are in the early stages. Researchers are often working under the radar, but still showing effective results with those already struggling with their brain health.

My father and I decided to take our own steps – together – to attempt to keep the onset of his disease in check and to search the world for the latest research. From scouring scientific journals, I have become aware that the medical profession's pharmaceutical options appear to be failing their trials, one by one, so I made the decision to turn in a non-invasive complementary direction instead.

There are myriad research papers showing the efficacy of herbal remedies and nutritional supplements as treatment for a wide range of ills – mental and physical. Many show that natural treatments can work just as well as pharmaceutical options. Some even anecdotally 'curing' officially 'incurable' diseases – although these are often attacked and shut down by corporate interests that have no intention of letting the majority of us be 'healed'. How much more profitable to keep 'managing' disease by medicating it instead of 'curing' it once and for all.

There is a wealth of new evidence on the phenomenon of 'epigenetics' – an area of work that looks at the way the expression of our DNA changes constantly depending on our brain's perception of, and response to, its environment, along with our ever-increasing understanding of the brain's plasticity. Epigenetics is revealing the mechanisms that explain how everything we do and are exposed to impacts on our brains.

A word of caution though, it's important to be mindful of the fact that a lack of research doesn't mean something doesn't work. Scientific research may give you confidence, but it often takes years, if not decades, to emerge into public view. If there is little profit to be made, corporate agendas may block the development, particularly of natural, non-invasive methods of healing because they are often not patentable. If large corporate funders can see no profit in such research, it is either unlikely to be funded, or any successes are rapidly buried.

Back to my father

We came to the conclusion that doing something had to be better than doing nothing but wait for the tide of forgetfulness to overwhelm him. And he has been brilliant, solidly supported by my stepmother every step of the way. First, we worked on his nutrition. We cut out everything that science shows has a negative effect on the brain. He stuck to his 'brain diet' (which I share with you in Chapter 7) religiously, and it gave him both hope and a structure. Each and every meal was scientifically proven to be able to improve his neuronal and mitochondrial strength and boost his mind.

Every therapy or supplement I researched that had substantial evidence of a positive effect on the brain, whether scientific or anecdotal, was added to his daily programme. He has enthusiastically done whatever it took – whether it was for an hour or a few minutes. He has taken part in trials in Canada looking at the effects of light therapy on the brain. We imported nutritional supplements from the US and silica-rich aluminium-removing water from Malaysia[2]. And we have tested his bloods and urine before and after each new element was introduced. Encouraged by every positive change, my father has become more confident that he might improve. With every mouthful that he eats, supplement he swallows, or potion that he drinks, he feels he is playing a part in his own recovery and taking back control of his health.

Looking at the wider audience

In the wake of my father's diagnosis, I began talking to people about dementia, and I noticed that much of the time a general air of despair accompanied it. There was a worrying dismissal from some quarters in response to my suggestions for what might help. I would tell my friends about a fascinating study on the effects of mindfulness on dementia, or the benefits of upping their intake of oily fish, for example, but much of this fell on stony ground. In most cases, my friends' scepticism had been stoked by their family doctor and other medical doctors' lack of awareness of research or anecdotal positive evidence on alternative treatments and lifestyle approaches.

I was struck, again and again, by an almost wilful rubbishing of alternative approaches. They seemed to come from a position of learned helplessness – drug treatments are too often presented as the only credible option. What particularly saddened me was that the dismissals mainly came from people who were already dealing with the early stages of dementia – they were in the trenches. But, even those whose brains seemed to be functioning fairly normally (although 'normal' for many people includes low-level anxiety, depression and brain fog), were, for the most part, equally disinterested.

I was repeatedly told that declining brain function: 'is just a normal part of getting older', 'it happens to us all', or 'there's nothing you can do about it'. But none of these statements is true. We have all met those vibrant, clear thinking 100-year olds, whose minds seem as sharp now as they were decades ago.

I kept wondering: what makes some people keep their brains and others lose theirs? Is it really just a question of genetics? The answer, quite simply, is – no, it isn't. Epigenetics has forced us all to reassess that idea. Look to your family past – how many of your great-grandparents succumbed to dementia – you will probably find it was the exception rather than the rule. So, what has changed? Granted, we are, for the most part, living for longer. But I believe it is in an analysis of the environment rather than the genes alone where you may find the answer. Today we live extremely sedentary lives, eat an unbalanced diet high in processed foods, sugars and animal products. We exist in a soup of electromagnetic frequencies, and drink and bathe in chemically treated water. Dangerously high levels of pollutants from transport and farming fill the air we breathe. The brain is a sensitive organ, and of course all of these environmental factors influence it.

How to start your journey of change

Perhaps I shouldn't have been surprised by the lack of engagement most of us have about thinking outside the box when it comes to the brain. The science behind our understanding of the brain's remarkable responsiveness to lifestyle and behavioural change is still relatively new. Most of us just haven't seen the memo yet.

If you're nodding your head with 'that's true of me' recognition, read on as I'd like to explore the importance of the latest scientific discoveries with you, and set them in context of our understanding of how our brains work. I'm hoping it might nudge you to shake up your thinking on what's possible.

I'll explain why current advances in neuroscience are so significant for anyone wanting to take a proactive approach to their brain health and function. I'm not talking specifically here about staving off dementia. I'm talking about improving your cognitive edge and enhancing your ability to harness the full power of your brainpower: memory, executive function (high level, complex and analytical thinking), as well as your emotional regulation, mood and energy. But everyone is different and so are the issues that affect them.

I have written this book to help you to take a more hopeful, empowering approach to your own mental health and brainpower. Most of the readily available approaches – drug therapies and long-term psychotherapy – are inadequate. The former is risky, and in many cases treats the symptoms rather than the causes of problems, and the latter is costly, very time-consuming and can be somewhat hit-and-miss in terms of its efficacy and availability.

I am going to show you how to take back control of your brain in three simple stages: first, unburden your brain, then repair it, and finally, boost it. Everything in this book is focused and evidence-based. I look at a range of possible interventions, many of which are lifestyle changes entirely within your control.

My research takes full advantage of the advances in neuroscience and the wide range of complementary health approaches that can help you. In writing it I have drawn on my 30 years' experience as a health advocate, from setting up Breast Cancer Haven all those years ago, to my health blog, www.reboothealth. co.uk. The more I've learned, the more passionate I've become about the potential we all have to take every aspect of our health into our own hands. This is nowhere truer than it is of the brain. And you can start on your journey today. Your reward will be to boost your brain function, improve your mental health and combat age-related cognitive decline.

Good luck with your journey, and let me know how you get on.

Sara

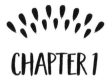

CHAPTER 1

ABOUT THE BRAIN

'It's now clear that many of our most sophisticated abilities are made possible not by specialist brain areas dedicated to specific tasks, but by lightning-fast coordination between areas that control more general tasks, such as movement and hearing.'

GEOFF WATTS, AUTHOR AND LEADERSHIP COACH

Before we go any further, let's start by looking at the brain and the nervous system as this will help you understand some of the terms I use in the book as well as why the techniques and therapies I have written about can help you.

Put simply, the brain, made up of billions of nerve cells, or neurons, is the centre of our thoughts, the interpreter of our external environment, and the origin of every bodily function and movement. It is the control centre of the central nervous system, which comprises the brain and the spinal cord that extends from its base. The peripheral nervous system is a network of nerve cells and fibres that link the brain and spinal cord with every part of the body. An autonomic nervous system, also under the control of the brain and its chemical messengers, controls essential body systems like breathing, heart rate and digestion.

Neurons each consist of a cell body with branching arms, called dendrites, that act like antennae and pick up messages. Axóns are similarly branching arms that carry messages away from the cell body. Impulses travel from neuron to neuron, from the axon of one cell to the dendrites of another, by crossing over a tiny gap between the two nerve cells called a synapse. Chemical messengers called neurotransmitters allow the electrical impulses to cross the gap.

The brain itself is made up of several different sections each with a separate function. There are three principal areas: the forebrain, the mid brain, and the hind brain, but these sections all work as part of the whole, as constantly firing neural pathways connect the different brain zones together. It's like a complex road network. Every part is located and has a name, but while it all works together as a whole, each section is also used in a wide variety of ways, all the time.

I will go into this in more detail in the second part of this chapter. First, I want to look at the recent developments in the study of the brain and nervous system – neuroscience – which go some way to explain the programme I have set out in this book.

The new science of neuroplasticity

'The discovery of neuroplasticity is the discovery that our brains can change their structure and function through mental experience alone.'

NORMAN DOIDGE, PSYCHIATRIST, PSYCHOANALYST AND AUTHOR

To understand the latest research developments, it's helpful to take stock of how far science has come. In Ancient Times natural philosophers focused purely on anatomy, and learning about the precise structure of the brain. Leonardo da Vinci's remarkable 15th-century anatomical drawings, for example, are still as exact and accurate as any images we see on the brain scanning machines of today.

Attention later shifted to understanding brain function. Towards the end of the 19th century, the concept of psychology emerged, under the aegis of the two foremost proponents of this new science, Sigmund Freud and Carl Jung. And by the end of the 20th century, psychology had grown into 53 main branches or 'schools', and from that developed more than 160 types, or approaches, of psychotherapy. In a way these different schools of thought are similar to a series of different religions, each with their independent followers and varying theories. But they are descriptive, not explanatory, ways of trying to understand how the brain works.

Nowadays, research is looking at how brain function and structure work together across the brain's myriad of differentiated parts and systems. This work has become even more urgent since the recent discovery that Freud turns out to have been what could effectively be described as a fraud, as his great cases are based on what he hoped was happening, not actual observation of events.[11] It is important to establish a clearer and more cohesive way of understanding and working with the brain going forwards, to unite the different theories and practices in a coherent science based on replicable experiments.

We know that psychology and psychiatry have made assumptions, then assumed they are true. Today's neuroscientists have demonstrated that, although some of them are valid, many of them are not. However, much of what began as theory and observation has subsequently gained clinical credence, as scientific discoveries shed new light on what dysfunctional and optimal brain function actually looks like. Neuroscience has confirmed what we already suspected about attachment theory and the origins of a wide range of psychiatric problems from depression to psychopathy. But until now, no commonly acknowledged science of the mind or behaviour has been developed – but the hope is that a clearer and more reliable picture is beginning to emerge.

Changing and adapting to behaviour and environment

You've probably heard the computing metaphor used in relation to your brain – that your mind, the software, lives in your brain, the hardware. But latest developments in neuroscience reveal this is not only somewhat simplistic but also inaccurate. To stretch the metaphor into something more useful, it has been discovered that even with short-term interventions, it's possible to change the 'hardware' of your brain by changing the way you use its 'software', and, better still, the latest brain scans show that the two are symbiotic. We can now 'see' that the 'hardware' or wiring pathways, dominant in grey matter, and cortical folding (see page 19), are constantly changing and adapting in response to new experiences, behaviours and environmental factors. This ability to change is known as neuroplasticity. The ever-increasing understanding of neuroplasticity shows us that our thoughts quite literally 'shape' our brains, just as much as our brains direct our thoughts.

A dizzying cocktail of factors constantly influences the physical brain. And, through iterative exposure, behavioural practice and habitual re-experiencing, our brain pathways actually change. The more dominant and deeply ingrained particular pathways become (through repeated activation), the more we will default to them. The brain's plasticity means we can deliberately direct the development of optimal thinking and our emotions and tap into its potential for change in ways not thought possible even 20 years ago.

An understanding of neuroplasticity has profound and positive implications for anyone interested in personal growth and the desire to make positive changes; it clearly demonstrates that you most certainly can teach old dogs new tricks – though they do have to want to learn them.

The golden age of neuroscience is now

In the past 30 years, neuroscience has really exploded thanks to the advent of sophisticated brain scanning technology, known as functional magnetic resonance imaging, or fMRI, which allows us to actually see the changes taking place in the brain. Theories are being proven and adapted as a result of careful observation of what is happening inside healthy brains, moment by moment, because neuroimaging shows precisely which parts of the brain light up when different responses occur. The new technology has led to huge leaps in the understanding of how much more the brain 'knows'. It has become clear that we are not rational beings, but rationalising beings. Our brains have decided what we are going to do before we know about it. Our thinking tries to make sense of what has already happened, but the brain is streets ahead of us in communicating, via the thoughts, feelings and behaviours we experience. Scientists can now see how trauma impacts on the brain, how our lifestyle and environment influence our thinking, and how utterly remarkable the brain's potential for regeneration and improvement is.

New technology is also opening up new possibilities for the 'mapping' of the brain's neural pathways and connections. Through experience, neurons can grow new branches, and synapses connecting neurons can grow, or shrink. The neuroscientist Professor Sebastian Seung, based at Princeton University, USA, is one of the leading lights in the new field, called 'Connectonomics'. Seung fuses neuroscience, physics and bioinformatics to map the brain in all its complexity. Using cutting-edge technology, his work is untangling the brain's complex wiring to better understand it.

Up to now research has focused on damaged and dysfunctional brains. With fMRI we can physically see both the changes resulting from injury and sickness, and those that take place in healthy, high-functioning brains. This is helping us gain an understanding not only of what brain optimisation 'looks' like, but the contributing factors that create it. The future will be about being able to direct the brain very precisely.

Advances in brain scanning have also forced the medical establishment to open its mind to alternative approaches to improving mental health and function. Research around practices once deemed esoteric, such as meditation, is forcing clinicians to challenge outdated assumptions about what has been considered 'out-there' in the past. Through the latest technology, science can observe physical changes in the brain as they happen, which will provide an insight into what really works, for example how long and how often we should practice mindfulness, or exercise, to gain any benefit. With that information it should be possible to come up with evidence-backed brain-boosting plans, including lifestyle changes and the adoption of key habits and daily behaviours.

The physiology of the brain

The main part of your brain – the wrinkly, folded (cortical folds), walnut-like grey matter – is divided into two almost identical cerebral hemispheres, each a mirror image of the other, which together make up about 85 per cent of the organ. Each hemisphere is split into four lobes (frontal, parietal, temporal and occipital), each with a different function, and covered by the neocortex, an outer covering that is made up of six thinner layers containing nerve cells and holding connectors that link it to other parts of the brain and the nervous system. The neocortex, also known as the thinking brain, is what makes us human. It enables us to plan and think logically and strategically. It is also the seat of consciousness, and of personality, as well as being responsible for fine-tuning movement.

Two other very important parts of the brain are the central limbic system and the brainstem at its base. The limbic system, also known as the mammalian brain, deals with feelings, memories and arousal. It comprises the amygdala, hippocampus, thalamus, hypothalamus, basal ganglia and cingulate cortex, located on both sides of the thalamus. The almond-shaped amygdala, which monitors the environment and connects it to the emotional system, is responsible for your 'fight–flight' threat response as well as falling in love. The brain stem, or reptilian brain, connects the brain to the central nervous system, via the spinal cord, and is the 'lowest' and most primitive region, common to all mammals and reptiles. It is responsible for basic survival functions, including eating, breathing and regulating your heart rate.

The diagrams opposite give you an idea of the shape and structure of the brain and will be useful to return to as you work through the book. See also the chart on page 20–21 for more on which part of the brain is responsible for which functions.

The anatomy of the brain

Complete brain

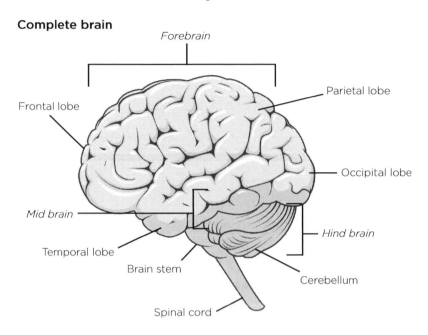

Forebrain

Frontal lobe
Parietal lobe
Occipital lobe
Mid brain
Hind brain
Temporal lobe
Brain stem
Cerebellum
Spinal cord

Cross section

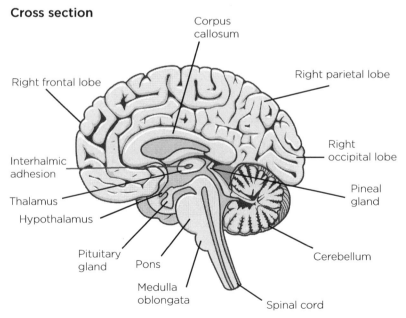

Corpus callosum
Right parietal lobe
Right frontal lobe
Right occipital lobe
Interhalmic adhesion
Pineal gland
Thalamus
Hypothalamus
Pituitary gland
Pons
Cerebellum
Medulla oblongata
Spinal cord

Main section	Subsection	Responsible for
Forebrain (prosencephalon), comprises the cerebrum, or telencephalon, and the cerebral cortex, six layers of different brain cells that lie directly underneath the skull. There are two hemispheres, right and left, and the corpus callosum runs between them, allowing them to communicate. Underneath are the basal ganglia. In the centre of the cerebrum sits the diencephalon – the thalamus, hypothalamus, subthalamus and epithalamus (which includes the pineal gland).	**Frontal lobe**, or cortex	Emotions becoming conscious, decision making, concentration, reasoning, creative thinking, language, information processing. Also controls movement, planning ahead, judgement, emotional expression, attention span, motivation, memory, inhibition, feeling, recall
	Parietal lobe, or cortex sits across the top and down the sides of your brain in the middle of your head	Association between senses, spatial awareness, touch, and awareness of time and space
	Occipital lobe, or cortex, sits at the back of the brain	Vision
	Temporal lobe, or cortex, sits on each side of your skull near your temples	Hearing, memory, learning, language, emotion, speech
	Corpus callosum	Connecting the left and right cerebral cortices
	Basal ganglia, the brain's pleasure centre	Dopamine-releasing neurons, habit forming, emotion processing, motivation and reward. Is also in charge of movement decisions
	Amygdala	Makes new neurons, attaches emotional content to memories, decides emotional response to feelings and the environment. It only stores memories that have strong emotional meaning
	Hippocampus	Long-term memory. It receives sensory data and integrates it into a single experience. Also responsible for spatial orientation, and is key for learning new things
	Thalamus, two lobes of grey matter that sit on top of the brainstem	Coordinator of all information coming into the brain. Processes sensory information and controls sleep and alertness. Thought to control and create consciousness

Hypothalamus	Regulates internal systems such as blood pressure and body temperature and connects autonomic, hormonal and visceral nervous and motor systems.
Pituitary gland	Hormone production and releases to thyroid and adrenal glands, ovaries and testes
Epithalamus, which includes the pineal gland a tiny, pine-cone like organ about the length of a grain of rice, is tucked between the lobes of the thalamus	Producing melatonin, and regulating hormones, circadian rhythms and the sleep-wake cycle
Subthalamus	Motor function
Cingulate cortex lies along midline of brain	Regulating emotions and pain and links behaviour outcomes to repeat responses
Insula	Perception of visceral responses such as heart rate, activity in gut, blood pressure

Mid brain (mesencephalon) is a connection point between the brain and the spinal cord – the information superhighway. There are three main parts – the tectum, the tegmentum and the cerebral peduncles.

Tectum	Visual and hearing maps of the world as well as visual/hearing signals and reflexes
Tegmentum, includes the cerebral aqueduct	Contains serotonin and dopamine producing neurons. Has a high concentration of endorphins. Suppresses pain, raises alertness, and coordinates movement
Cerebral penduncles	Body coordination – it carries motor signals from the brain to muscles

Hind brain (metencephalon) includes most of the brainstem

Pons (from Latin, meaning bridge)	Sleep, breathing, swallowing, body functions and bladder control, eye movement, sensation and posture
Medulla oblongata	Respiration and heart rhythms
Cerebellum	Movement, control, motor learning, balance, emotion and learning, posture, abstract reasoning, language control, precision. Determines your ability to drive a car, tie your shoelace or hit a ball.

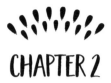

CHAPTER 2

YOUR BRAIN BASELINE

*'Humans do use 100 per cent of their brains over
the course of a day. They just don't use every
section at once.'*

JOHN HENLEY, NEUROLOGIST

Mapping your brain

To begin this process you need to understand your own brain
health and the factors that affect it. So where should you
start? Unfortunately, I can't offer you a functional magnetic
resonance image (fMRI) of your brain, but I have prepared a brain
baseline questionnaire that can help you identify the range of
stressors that your brain might be susceptible to. Then as you work
through the book, take the appropriate steps to support better brain
function and brain health, using the advice I share in 'Action Plans' at
each and every stage.

First, I want to make you aware of how many different external
and internal forces can shape the function of your brain – it's

important to understand from the outset that these won't be the same for everybody, any more than the solutions will be.

But before looking at the longer questionnaire, you can rate your brain energy and function by answering the three simple questions below – and I will ask you to do this again at the end of the book.

1.   On a scale of 1 to 10, where 1 equals exhausted and foggy headed, and 10 is able to think on your feet, feeling energised and well rested, how do you rate your mental energy?

2.   On a scale of 1 to 10, where 1 equals very depressed, and 10 is joyful, how do you rate your mood?

3.   On a scale of 1 to 10, where 1 equals unable to form clear thoughts, and 10 is able to harness your full brain power to think with clarity and decisiveness, how do you rate your mental clarity?

The brain baseline questionnaire

Stress-check your own brain. The stressors that can impact it may be environmental (air pollution, chemicals in the water or your home), physical (spinal misalignment, concussion, high cholesterol, gut microbiome problems, a build-up of toxic metals), habit-based (sedentary lifestyle, commuting), health-based (diet, hydration), and emotional (divorce, anxiety, bereavement). Each of these factors cause inflammation in the brain which, long term, contributes to cognitive impairment and the decline of brain function and mental health. Before you start, it's important to make it clear that because the risk factors are so varied and interconnected, it is difficult to be precise about them all – you cannot crunch data on the specifics of your neighbourhood, home, daily routine, and so on. While it's impossible to turn this questionnaire into a tidy quiz with a scientific 'score' that tells you the exact degree of stress your brain is under, it can give you a picture of the problem areas. The checklists, all backed by published studies and data (you'll find the references at the back of the book), provide a starting point that can get you thinking about what you can do to reduce potential damage to your brain and restrict its impairment by factors that are within your control.

Work through each section and give yourself one point for any of the statements that you answer positively or nothing for a negative answer – but deduct one if you see '-1' next to the question as these are the things that are already helping to protect your brain. The overall score for each section will highlight the areas where a change may help. The actions that arise out of the quiz are self-evident. Starting today, prioritise all the positive things you can do to avoid, cut out or change the stressors.

Part 1: Environmental stressors

Small particulate matter from air pollution and nitrous oxide from traffic is known to impact on brain function, so consider where you live, where you walk and how you travel. Similarly, exposure to chemicals at work, on nearby farms (or indirect exposure if you live with somebody who works with chemicals), could be affecting you. Household mould, which is hugely common, is another often neglected cause of neurological symptoms, and one that it's relatively easy to treat. On top of all this, everything from your smart utilities meter to hours spent at your computer or using your mobile phone may be having an impact on your brain too.

- Do you live within 500m ($^1/_3$ mile) of heavy traffic?[1] ....

- Do you live within 5km (3 miles)[2] of factory pollution?[3] ....

- Do you live within 400m ($^1/_4$ mile) of a mobile phone tower? [4] If you live in the US, visit www.antennasearch.com to find out where your nearest tower is.

  ....

- Do you live within 750m ($^1/_2$ mile) of crop spraying?[5]...............

- Do you live in a 'green' neighbourhood, close to trees?[6] (score -1 if yes) ....

- Does anyone in your home work in agriculture, or in buildings where chemicals are present? ....

- Have you been exposed to chemicals in your current or past job?[7] ....

- Do you work with glues, solvents or paints?[8] ....

- Do you regularly smell any of the following on entering your house?
  Gas?[9] ....
  Mould?[10] ....

- Do you have copper water pipes in your house?.........................

- Are you aware of chemicals from furniture (new mattresses or sofas), or do you live in a new house, or in rooms freshly decorated with non-organic paints? [11]

  ....

- Do you spend 7 or more hours per day in front of a screen (include computer, TV, tablets and phones)?[12]..............................

- Do you regularly use hands-free (bluetooth) headphones with your mobile phone?[13]

  ....

- Do you have a smart meter for gas and/or electricity in your home, or does a close neighbour have one?[14] ....

- Do you work in an environment where you are exposed to breathing in heavy metals? ....
  If the answer is yes:
  Are you a dentist or dental assistant?[15] ....
  Do you work with phosphate fertilisers? ....
  Do you work in the plastic, paint or glass industry? ....
  Do you work with steel and metal machining or electrical and wiring components? ....

Part 2: Assess your habits

Every aspect of your daily routine, from commuting to exercise, sleep to daily meditation, and even having a pet, can have a profound impact on your brain and its ability to function. Changing these habits, or taking up new, healthier ones, is a way to take back control of the circumstances that impact on your cognitive ability, mood and the way your brain ages.

- Do you drive for more than 2 hours a day?[16] ....

- Do you walk or bike to work? (score -1 if yes)[17] ....

- Including time spent at work, commuting and at leisure, do you sit for an average of:
  Less than 4 hours a day? [18] (score -1 if yes) ....
  4–7 hours? ....
  7–10 hours? ....
  11 hours plus? ....

- Do you exercise so that you are out of breath for 2 hours a week (brisk walking counts)?[19] (-1 if yes) ....

- Do you practice meditation regularly? [20] (-1 if yes) ....

- Do you get 7–8 hours of good-quality sleep per night? [21] (-1 if yes, +1 if less than 7–8, as well as +1 if more than 9)...

- Do you exercise near busy roads regularly (including walking)?[22] ....

- Have you smoked cannabis regularly at any point in your life?[23] ....

Part 3: Diet, hydration, alcohol and smoking

There is such an abundance of information out there on healthy eating, alcohol and smoking, that it can almost take on the quality of white noise. It's all too easy to just get on with your life and zone it out, partly because there is so much of it, but also because of a lot of it appears contradictory. With this in mind, I've tried to keep this section of the quiz simple.

- Do you eat 1–4 portions or more of oily fish per week?[24] (-1 if yes) ....

- Do you eat meat?[25] ....

- Do you supplement with Vitamin D? (-1 if yes)[26] ....

- Do you take regular nutritional supplements? (-1 if yes)..........

- Do you drink more than 6 glasses of water per day? (-1 if yes)..

- Do you eat 3 or more portions per day or more of vegetables?[27] (-1 if yes)..

- Do you eat 3 or more pieces of fruit per day?[28] (-1 if yes) ....

- Do you consume more than 6 teaspoons of sugar (women) or more than 9 for men on an average day – don't forget to include hidden sugars?[29] ....

- Do you smoke?..

- Do you live with a smoker?...

- Do you drink more than 1 unit of alcohol per day?[30].................

Part 4: Look at your general health

There are plenty of simple ways to check your physical health. These following questions relate to brain health and function, as well as bodily health. Some of them are symptomatic of cognitive decline, but others simply demonstrate that your brain, like your body, is under increased stress as a result of your lifestyle, habits and environment.[31]

- Do you regularly get colds and flu?..

- Do you regularly visit an osteopath or chiropractor for back pain? (-1 if yes)..

- Have you ever suffered from concussion? ....

- Have you ever had whiplash? ....

- Do you take a daily probiotic? (-1 if yes)......................................

- Do you have mercury fillings, implants or root canals in your teeth?..

- Is your urine pale yellow in colour?[32] (-1 if yes; +1 if no)............

- Is your blood pressure too high? You can buy a blood pressure monitor online for under £15 or ask your GP to check it. The healthy range is 120/80–140/90 ....

- Do you have high cholesterol? (If your total reading is greater than 5, or between 4 and 5, you are at a high risk of heart disease)?[33]..

- Has your eyesight been becoming steadily worse despite the fact you are in your 60s or older and expected your vision to have settled after middle age?[34] ....

- Do you often appear puffy or bloated?[35] ....

- Have you taken antibiotics recently?[36] ....

Part 5: Your emotional wellbeing

Brain function has a huge emotional component, and emotional wellbeing feeds into a range of aspects of mental health and cognitive function. Asking yourself a few simple questions will help you to build a picture of your emotional wellbeing and consider the impact of this on your brain.

- Would you describe yourself as lonely?[37] ....

- Are you happily living with a partner?[38] (-1 if yes) ....

- Do you find fulfilment in your job? (-1 if yes) ....

- Do you have a difficult relationship in your life? ....

- Do you suffer from any of the following?[39]
  (score one point for each)
  Panic attacks ....
  Anxiety ....
  Depression ....

- Have you experienced long-term stress?[40] ....

- Is the stress in your life unpredictable, affecting you randomly in ways you cannot anticipate?[41] ....

- Do you regularly experience 'flow' where you lose yourself in an activity you love? (-1 if yes) ....

- Do you have a supportive social network?[42] (-1 if yes) ....

- Have you experienced any major traumatic emotional experiences, including the following, within the last year?[43] (score one point for each)

  - Divorce ....

  - Betrayal..

  - Bereavement...

  - Redundancy ....

  - Other..

Three keys to maintaining brain health

Where does it begin? Why do our brains struggle? Decline creeps up so slowly over decades that it's almost impossible to notice the difference, until one day your mind is no longer as acute as once it was. Manage the three fundamentals to brain health – first, keep your mitochondria numbers up, secondly, keep inflammation down and, thirdly, minimise the number of senescent cells (those that have stopped dividing and replicating, but also refuse to die) – and you are much of the way there. Each of these elements is interlinked, so the odds are that if you are affected by one, the others will also be an issue.

The first key: Your mitochondria

Mitochondria are the tiny batteries that power up your brain cells. They generate more than 90 per cent of the energy your body needs to live and your brain needs to function.

Mitochondria also dictate how rapidly – or slowly – you age. They need oxygen to survive and, because your oxygen levels fall over time (usually because of the stresses of everyday living such as an overload of environmental chemicals and toxins, electromagnetic fields/EMFs and poor diet), they weaken and reduce in number as you age. As mitochondria begin to mutate and stop working, so eventually do you.

Your mitochondria create free radicals that play an important part in the health of your immune system, attacking any invaders and helping to turn the air that you breathe and the food that you eat into energy. Stress, however, can cause them to produce too many free radicals, which can affect your DNA and cause brain cells to mutate and die. Radiation from mobile phones damages your mitochondria, and can damage your genes. The worse your lifestyle choices – eat too many unhealthy fried or fatty foods, drink too much alcohol and inhale too many pesticides, chemicals and tobacco – the higher the level of mitochondrial dysfunction.

Action plan

- **Adopt the mito food plan** This is an anti-inflammatory, gluten-free, high-quality fat, low-grain, low glycaemic diet that supports your mitochondria and improves their energy production. For advice check www.centerforfunctionalmedicine.com

- **Take pyrroloquinoline quinone (PQQ) supplements** PQQ increases your number of mitochondria, and improves their efficiency and is also thought to promote new neuronal growth. Combining it with coenzyme 10, CoQ10, (see Chapter 7) may lead to improved cognitive health and better memory.

- **Boost your oxygen levels** Surround yourself with oxygen-boosting plants such as the gerbera daisy, spider plant, Boston fern, snake plant or areca palm. Try yoga pranayama breathing. Supplement with Cellfood, a nutritional supplement scientifically proven to oxygenate your body efficiently. www.cellfood.co.uk

- **Take antioxidants** These will reduce the oxidative stress triggered when your free radical numbers rise. Minerals such as selenium, vitamins A, C and E, foods like blueberries, goji berries, pomegranates, and the supplement CoQ10 (see Chapter 7), are all good sources of antioxidants.

- **Sign up for a course of intermittent hypoxic hyperoxic therapy (IHHT)** This involves breathing in oxygen through a mask, but alternating low-oxygen air (hypoxic) with high-oxygen air (hyperoxic), to destroy old mitochondria and stimulate the development of new healthy ones in their place.

The second key: Inflammation

Inflammation, meaning 'in flames', literally means that your body is 'on fire' and indicates that there is severe irritation in your tissues and cells somewhere, often deep down, which may be accompanied by a raised body temperature. A raised temperature is simply a signal that your body is using its energy to fight something on your behalf – energy that could be better used elsewhere. You can see inflammation quite clearly if you look for it, for example, someone might have a slightly puffed face, or swollen wrists or ankles. Other signs of inflammation include aching joints and muscles, continual exhaustion, rashes or redness and brain fog.

Caused by poor eating habits, viral or bacterial overload, or extreme stress, inflammation is the starting point for many diseases. It is also linked to high cholesterol levels, which can lead to a build-up of fatty plaques in your arteries and in your brain. Over time, chronic inflammation can cause DNA damage, and trigger depression and cancer. Raised levels of inflammation in your brain increases production of amyloid proteins as a defence mechanism, which increases the risk of dementia.

Action plan

- **Ask your doctor for a C-reactive protein test** This is a test that measures the amount of inflammation in your body.

- **Take probiotics** Certain bacteria in the gut cause inflammation. By taking specific brain, or 'psycho', biotics, you can rebalance the microbiome in your gut and control inflammation levels.[44] (See also Reference section, page 266)

- **Supplement with curcumin** This is the active ingredient in turmeric and one of the most potent natural anti-inflammatory remedies. It works by reducing the production of cytokines, the molecules that trigger inflammation (see also Chapter 7).[45]

- **Add more ginger to your diet** Ginger switches off a signalling pathway that links inflammation with cancer and dementia. It also reduces the numbers of both cytokines and cyclooxygenase enzymes that increase inflammation.

- **Take herbal remedies** Devil's claw, turmeric (see curcumin, above) and willow bark are all natural remedies that reduce inflammation levels.

- **Supplement with BioBran** This is one of the fastest ways to boost your immune system and get inflammation in check. BioBran is a natural supplement made from rice bran broken down by the enzymes of shitake mushrooms and taking it daily will increase your natural killer (NK) cells by up to 300 per cent, B-cells by 250 per cent, and T-cells by 200 per cent within two to three weeks. www.healthy.co.uk

Peptide therapy – a brain medicine of the future?

Peptides are naturally occurring biological molecules. Brain peptides are 'brain foods' that slow down inflammation in the brain. They are tiny molecules used by the neurons to communicate with each other and include oxytocin, vasopressin, angiotensin, NCH and hypocretin. They need to be prescribed by a qualified doctor, so consult a trained medical practitioner for advice. The International Peptide Society, headed up by Dr William Seeds, is at the forefront of this developing science. www.peptidesociety.org

Some peptides can penetrate the blood–brain barrier to reduce inflammation and repair the immune system, while others work on synapse repair. Cerebral lysine, for example, repairs memory. A NAP peptide, recently developed by a doctor in Tel Aviv, Israel, has been shown to both protect and restore the microtubule network in the central nervous system, a transportation system within our nerve cells that carries messages and proteins from cell to cell, offering hope for neurological diseases such as Alzheimer's and Parkinson's. L-Serine stops the build-up of proteins in the brain and Thymosin Alpha 1 helps boost immunity and reduce inflammation.[46] Synapsin is a blend of peptides that can be used as a nasal spray to support cognitive function and develop new neuronal pathways and can help symptoms of dementia and Parkinson's. BPC-157 has been shown to reduce cell damage in the hippocampus of rats, protecting brain tissue.

LINX™ Alzheimer's-associated immune reactivity test

Although the field of medicine currently has no cure for dementia, natural approaches have been shown in repeated scientific studies to make a quantifiable difference. The LINX test looks at nearly 40 biomarkers in the brain to identify risk factors to neurological decline and Alzheimer's disease, many of which are years in the making. So, identifying any issues and intervening with natural methods long before they become a diagnosed condition seems a sensible approach. For example, some people have immune reactions to foods that have a similar molecular structure to amyloid beta, which creates antibodies that can cause the immune system to attack the amyloid beta. The test identifies elevated antibodies to these foods so that, if you have the antibodies, you can eliminate these foods from your diet to protect your brain. (Available from Health Natural – admin@robertjacobshealth.com)

The third key: Senescent cells

Statistics show that as you age, both your body and your brain progressively lose the ability to regenerate and repair themselves, a process known as senescence. Your immune system simply ages and as it does so there is a knock-on effect on the central nervous system and the brain: genes mutate; chromosomes are damaged; tissues, arteries and organs clog up; your energy-generating mitochondria start to fail and inflammation sets in. The end result is a fact of life – you become frail.

Frailty is caused by an increase in the number of cells that have stopped dividing and replicating themselves, but the cells also refuse to die – these are called senescent cells. Normally, a strong immune system could remove them by force, but as your immune system slows it fails to contain them and they 'go rogue', causing widespread inflammation and damage to the surrounding tissues, and give off chemical signals that convert nearby cells to the same senescent state. If you can increase the numbers of your B- and T-cells you can, to some degree, reverse this immune system collapse and slow the process of ageing – reinvigorating your brain in the process.

It is in the rapidly growing field of immunology that the solution to healthy brain ageing seems likely to be found as new treatments for neurodegenerative and neuropsychiatric disorders targeting age-linked inflammation emerge. At the Maharaj Institute of Immune Regenerative Medicine in Florida, USA, Dr Dipnarine Maharaj uses a sophisticated blood test that measures a wide range of blood parameters to establish precise immune senescence and inflammation levels (known as 'inflammaging').[47] Dr Maharaj has developed a treatment where inflammation and immune function in patients with neurological conditions such as multiple sclerosis, and Parkinson's, Alzheimer's and motor neurone (or ALS) diseases are corrected with the patients' own stem cells.[48] The Institute is also researching the use of stem-cell-mobilised plasma from donors aged 18 to 35 for the treatment of immune senescence associated frailty. Healthy young stem cells have been shown to rejuvenate older cells, restoring brain function in the process. In addition, the Maharaj Institute is offering to harvest and store healthy patients bone-marrow stem cells, for use later in life when they may need to decrease levels of inflammation and reboot their immune function to stave off frailty.

Action plan

- **Take BioBran supplements daily** Developed more than 20 years ago in Japan, BioBran is a natural supplement made from rice bran broken down by the enzymes of shitake mushrooms. Within two to three weeks, levels of NK cells have been shown to increase by up to 300 per cent, B-cells by 250 per cent, and T-cells by 200 per cent.

- **Take supplements that boost your circulating stem cells** Stem cells are neutral cells that can turn into any other type of cell, and mend whichever area of your body needs assistance. The polyphenols and antioxidants found in goji berries, pomegranates, green tea and blueberries can increase bone-marrow-derived stem cells.

- **Try intermittent fasting** In a 2017 study,[49] 100 participants fasted on five consecutive days each month, for three months. During the fasting they ate a plant-based diet of 800–1,100 calories, which both reduced inflammation and boosted circulating stem cells.

- **Increase exercise (see page 164-70)** Start doing High-intensity interval training (HIIT) as it increases the number of circulating stem cells and boosts your brain.[50] (See also Chapter 7.)

A warning about senolytic therapy

Some pharmaceutical companies are promoting senolytic therapy, which uses specially developed drugs intended to kill senescent cells, effectively allowing healthy cells to 'breathe' and function as they should. However, there is a fundamental problem with this. Destroying senescent cells simply speeds up the ageing process of any remaining cells, which have to divide to replace the removed cells. Studies show that, although there may be a temporary improvement, immediately afterwards there is an acceleration in the course of disease.

Telomeres and vitamin E – the key to anti-ageing

Telomeres are found at the end of each of your chromosomes. They hold them together, protecting them from damage and 'fraying' or sticking to one another, which could confuse genetic information. The longer they are, the more vibrant your health; conversely, shorter telomeres mean that you're likely to be more prone to chronic diseases and reduced life expectancy. Each time a cell divides, your telomeres shorten. If you take action to lengthen them, however, you can reverse the situation.

Vitamin E combines eight substances – four tocopherols and four telomere-boosting tocotrienols. The latter can cross the blood–brain barrier and are powerful telomere protectors and all four can lengthen them. The results of one Malaysian study showed that cells given gamma tocotrienol were not only protected from telomere shortening but that it also preserved telomerase (the enzyme that rebuilds your telomeres) activity in the cells. Hopefully within a few years, you should be able to rejuvenate your brain with a single injection of a natural protein. In the meantime, try the following action plan.

What you can do to help

- **Add tocotrienol-rich foods to your diet** The best source is annatto oil, from the Andean achiote tree, as it contains roughly 15mg per tablespoon, while palm oil has 8mg per tablespoon. You can also get tocotrienols from nuts and dark leafy greens; a handful of cashews, almonds or pistachios provides around 2mg and one serving of kale, broccoli or spinach has between 1mg and 2mg.

- **Take a tocotrienol supplement** You will need 50mg twice a day and it should be taken with a meal. Try Now Food's Gamma E Complex Advanced. www.uk.iherb.com

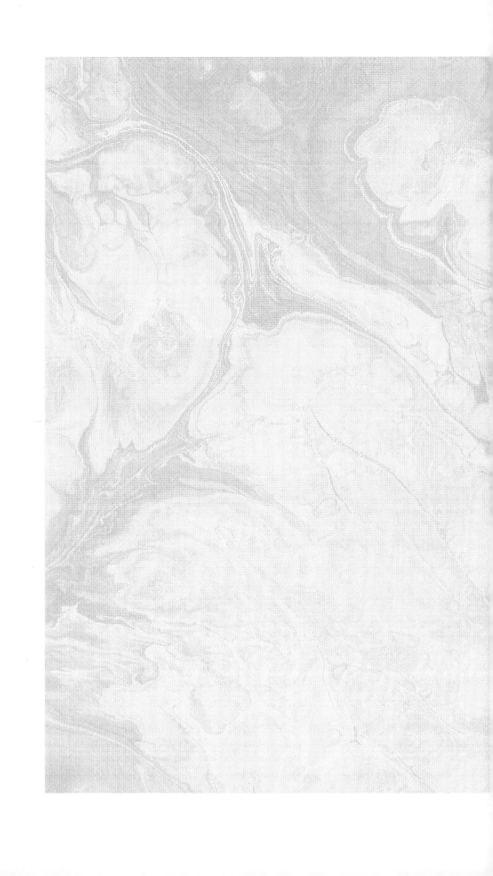

STEP ONE

—

UNBURDEN *Your* Brain

'Understanding your own anatomy and how it functions is crucial to changing your thinking and changing your life.'

TONI SORENSON

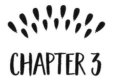

CHAPTER 3

TIME TO DETOX

'Because we cannot scrub our inner body we need to learn a few skills to help cleanse our tissues, organs and mind...'

SEBASTIAN POLE, MASTER HERBALIST

So many new and unnatural substances have been created in the last few decades it is no surprise that our brains and bodies struggle to keep up and acclimatise to them – we are bombarded by 1,000s of chemical toxins every day. Air pollution levels are rising to the point that many of us are inhaling air with many times higher levels of particulates than is considered safe. Our water contains carcinogenic substances and our food is no longer safe from genetic modification (GMO) and chemical interference. Synthetic fertilisers and pesticides are making the Earth – and ourselves – sick. In addition, our homes are built with products known to be carcinogenic – including lead, PVC, creosote, flame-retardant chemicals, and the volatile organic compounds (VOCs) found in solvents, paints and plastic coatings. We then fill our homes with furniture made from similarly harmful toxic products and, to cap it all off, we clean them (and ourselves) with chemical-laden substances.

There are more than 3,000 different chemicals used to make cleaning products and toiletries, make-up, hair spray, sun creams, body lotions, perfume, and shower and bath gels. We breathe them in and rub them into our skin. Over time they build up in the body, hampering its ability to rid itself of the unwanted synthetic chemical by-products.[1] Residues from plastics in bottles, pesticides and detergents are an obvious example – they mimic hormones, blocking oestrogen or progesterone and wreak havoc with your adrenal and thyroid glands.[2] Little wonder then that your body is poorly equipped to deal with the chemical onslaught, and struggles to deal with a toxic overload that simply didn't exist in days gone by. On top of all that, your body has to adapt to a world of increased and unnatural frequencies and vibrations, all of which impact in invisible ways. We exist in an electromagnetic 'soup', drowning in smartphones, computers, tablets, routers, wearable tech, smart meters and now, white goods connected to the 'internet of things'. We are also surrounded by mobile phone masts and Wi-Fi, which constantly zap us with electrical frequencies that have been shown to have an adverse effect on human cells – take a look at the studies I referenced in the brain baseline questionnaire for the low-down. All of this extra stimulation interferes with our concentration, memory and ability to think laterally and creatively.

The answer is detox...

If your environment is making you ill, you need to reduce the effects of everyday pollution by calling on your own in-built 'rubbish removers' to lighten your brain's load. Detox is not a fluffy lifestyle choice anymore; it's become a necessity.

The aim of detoxing is to support your body's naturally efficient waste disposal systems: your skin, lungs, liver, kidneys, colon and lymphatic system. Each plays its own part in disposing of harmful 'stuff' via your sweat, breathing, urine, bowels, and for women, your monthly period. But, like your brain, the organs behind these processes may be similarly overloaded by the pollutants of everyday living. However, clean them up and they will work for you at full force – the benefit will be nothing short of a mental and physical power-up.

The four-step brain detox

The simple fact, though, is that your body isn't equipped to rid itself of today's overload of toxins by itself – it needs additional assistance from you. I use the terms toxic and toxins here to relate to anything – chemical, electromagnetic or 'other' – that builds up in the body and brain and hampers your ability to function optimally.

When you understand what is affecting you on a day-to-day basis, and how your total 'toxin load' may be affecting your brain, you can take the steps necessary to reduce it. So, here goes...

1. Join the toxic dots

Go back to the results from your brain–baseline quiz in Chapter 2. What did it tell you about the particular cocktail of toxic stress your brain and body are subject to? Run through your list of brain-related symptoms and think about any toxic contributors that could be to blame. What are your symptoms? When did they start? Consider everything – even seemingly insignificant chemical changes. Did it start when you changed to a new brand of soap powder, or put that chemical fragrance plug-in in your bedroom? Or was it starting a new job involving chemicals or pesticides? Did you start using a Wi-Fi booster, or increase the number of devices in your house? And rate the severity of any symptoms (particularly those that are hard to quantify, such as brain fog). It can be difficult to remember quite how bad those symptoms felt at the beginning when you are several months down the line of your brain recovery.

2. Identify toxins that you may be coming into contact with day-to-day

Go through your house with a proverbial fine-toothed comb. Look at the products you use in the bathroom. Read the labels on your toothpaste and your shampoos; you'll probably be amazed at how many incomprehensible words you find in the small print. If you can't understand what it says, it is not likely to be a natural substance – maybe consider buying organic next time. Do the same for the stuff under your kitchen sink, or in the cleaning cupboard.

Next think about electromagnetic field (EMF) exposure. Look around the home to see where your router is and where you have your devices. Also look at where you live in relation to mobile phone towers and electricity pylons. Do the same for pollution – when are the pollution levels at their highest during the day, and when do you have your doors and windows open? Does it coincide? Conversely, if you keep your doors and windows closed day and night, you will need regular fresh air to disperse the indoor build-up of chemicals (just do it at times when air pollution is low).

3. Cut out as many toxins from your life as is practically possible

- Eat organic (especially pesticide-free) where you can (see also Chapter 7).

- Drink filtered rather than tap water – if you buy water from the supermarket choose glass bottles rather than plastic.

- Avoid air pollution wherever feasible. Avoid busy main roads – take the back roads to the shops. Stay on the inside of pavements, away from the traffic. Don't walk in the countryside when crops and fields are being sprayed. Invest in air purifying technology for your home and car.

- Swap synthetic sheets and clothes for organic, natural fibres – and wash them before you use them.

- Get out and exercise more, ideally somewhere green. This will oxygenate your blood and boost your immune system. If you live in a city, exercise away from busy roads.

- Buy a magnetic field meter to test the electromagnetic waves in your house and avoid sleeping, sitting or working in areas with high readings. The Gauss machine is not expensive.

4. Clean up your organs

Healthy organs are key to a healthy brain. Schedule a regular detox of the organs that help with elimination – your skin, lungs, liver, colon, kidneys, and lymph glands – to help them help your body to process the overload of environmental toxins (see below). For more on dietary advice, see Chapter 7.

Look after your skin

The skin is often overlooked as a means of eliminating toxins, yet it is porous, and in a matter of seconds takes in what you put on it. This is picked up by your blood and carried all around your body and ultimately up into your brain.

Think about the clothes you wear day in day out. Are they synthetic and sprayed with chemicals that leach into your body? Any item of clothing that is not organic is likely to have been sprayed with solvents, acids, dyes and flame retardants that have been proven by research to be carcinogenic. Swap to organic cotton, silk, linen, hemp, wool, flax or linen where you can, and even then wash it before you first wear it.

What about the sheets, pillowcases and pillows you sleep on each and every night – so close to your brain? Or the pollutants in your mattress that you inhale unknowingly as you sleep? Memory foam is often full of noxious gases – do you know how they may be affecting your brain? Sleep should be a time for your brain to renew and repair, not struggle to fend off a wave of invisible toxins.

Have you stopped to think about contaminants in the water that you shower in? Most tap water contains small amounts of toxic chemicals like fluoride, arsenic, chlorine, metals and nitrates and other cancer-causing substances, which have been shown to be the cause of many health problems. What is in the water goes into your body via your skin. It is absorbed in tiny quantities, but over time, the impact is worth thinking about.

Action plan

- **Try dry skin brushing** Give your skin a quick scrub with a long-handled brush each morning before you shower. This will rid it of the toxins you sweated out each night and stimulate your lymph and blood circulation.

- **Get sweaty** Take exercise that makes you sweat as sweating eliminates toxins. Stretching and Pilates are simply not enough. Go for a 5km (3 mile) run, join an aerobics class, get skipping or do push ups in the park till you glow. A session in a sauna, hot tub or steam room is another way to speed up elimination through sweating. Fit regular sessions into your schedule – but always remembering to replace lost fluids by drinking 2 litres (4 pints) of water (toxin-free) during and afterwards.

- **Fit a full-house water filter** Make sure you are bathing in, cooking with and drinking toxin-free water.

Did you know:
How much of your body is water?

After oxygen, water is your body's most important nutrient so it is vital to keep drinking it regularly throughout the day. On average your body is 60 per cent water – the brain is 73 per cent water, muscles are 79 per cent, blood is 90 per cent, and your other organs range from 70 to 90 per cent. Water flushes toxins out of all your body cells, including your brain, and excretes them via your urine. If your body loses more fluid than you take in (dehydration) it can affect body function. Even mild dehydration has been shown to have a negative effect on your brain function.

Clear your lungs

Your lungs are your body's air purifiers. They act as filters, removing the dust and dirt and pollution from the 11,000 litres of air that you breathe daily. They pick up oxygen from the air that you breathe in and deliver it to your bloodstream, and remove carbon dioxide and other waste products from your body when you breathe out. Have you noticed that if you walk or cycle through a car-congested city or town, you will arrive at your destination covered in small black particles all over your skin and your clothes? That's what your lungs have to deal with on a daily basis, which is why you often cough up mucus to lighten their load.

The impact of pollution on the brain is currently the focus of a number of scientific studies. A study in Beijing, China, has shown that air pollution has a negative impact on the brain's white matter,[3] and that consistent exposure negatively impacts on intelligence, and language processing in particular. Men seem to be disproportionately impacted, perhaps because women's brains have more white matter.

Air pollution is hard to avoid. There are more than 85,000 'permitted' chemicals in our world nowadays and the air that we breathe is full of particulates that cause disease (in the UK alone, an estimated 80,000 people die from air pollution every year). One study found that in some places on the London Underground air pollution was up to 30 times higher than on busy roads above. Even if you live in the countryside and may think you are safe, the pesticides and chemical sprays used by farmers travel with the wind.

Studies have shown that these chemicals leave their residue in your tissues and your fat. Although it can take years or even decades to trigger the cellular changes that cause disease, there's little doubt that they do. Farm and industrial workers are often at the extreme end of the exposure scale, but the frequent court cases involving workers who report cancers, increased incidence of degenerative brain conditions, and birth defects are proof enough that the human body is vulnerable to chemical interference.

In addition, as we age, our cells begin to process oxygen less efficiently, leaving the mitochondria to struggle to produce the energy we need each day, and over time depleting the oxygen levels in the blood. However, boost your body's cells with high-quality oxygen, and you will reboot both your physical body, your energy levels, and your brain function.

Long-term effects of polluted air

The World Health Organisation estimates that around 4.2 million deaths globally can be linked to air pollution annually. Nine out of 10 of us breathe in polluted air every day – we just can't see the pollutants. Nitrogen oxide, from traffic fumes, causes oxidative stress, but the greatest damage comes from the PM2.5 particulates coming out of our car engines, wood smoke and coal fires. A recent study tracked the progress of identically sized gold particulates breathed in via the nose. It found that the gold penetrated every part of the body, including the brain, and the 'second (gut) brain' (see Chapter 8), affecting its microbiome. There is currently no researched method of clearing these pollutants. Some may be released via urine, but in general, levels of air pollutants simply accumulate. Is this perhaps a cause of the rapid rise in neurological conditions like autism, attention deficit hyperactivity disorder ADHD, dementia, Parkinson's disease and multiple sclerosis?

Action plan

● **Find out about the pollution levels in your surroundings**
Experiment with Plume lab's 'Flow' machine, a tiny device
that you strap to your belt or your bag which measures how
clean – or not – the air that you breathe really is. Even moving
a few feet away from the road edge of the pavement can
dramatically improve the readings. Assess the pollutant levels
inside your living or working space, too. Without accurate
measurements, it is difficult to manage or control the purity
of your air. The uHoo is an inside air monitor that covers nine
different parameters. www.uhooair.co.uk

● **Boost the levels of oxygen in your blood** Try yoga breathing
exercises – the meditations in the daily practices described
in Chapter 9 provide a great opportunity to focus on your
breaths.

● **Wear a good-quality air filtration mask in busy traffic** Wear
a mask when you are driving, cycling or on foot. A great one
is the R-Pur, made by a French tech company, which can
filter even the tiniest micro-particulates: most masks filter to
PM2.5, but this one filters particles 60 times smaller – PM
0.04. It picks up toxic particles, pollen, viruses, bacteria and
diesel exhaust particles. www.r-Pur.com

● **Buy an air filtration system** This can clean up the air in your
home.

● **Clean up pollution levels inside your car** These are often up
to 21 per cent higher than the levels of the air outside and
nitrogen dioxide levels in particular can be up to 10 times the
legal limit. Fit an air purifier such as the Airbubbl, the only
one that removes over 95 per cent of the particulates, gases
and nitrogen dioxide from inside your car. Airbubbl.com

- **Invest in a ClearO2 can** This is an oxygen cannister that you can buy for less than £20. Keep one at home and boost your oxygen levels by taking 8–10 inhalations a day. Clearo2.com
- **Sign up for a few sessions in a pressurised hyperbaric chamber** Breathing oxygen in through a nasal canula at pressure floods your bloodstream with pure oxygen. Your body can take in 95 per cent of the oxygen, which penetrates deep into your cells, including your brain and your nervous system. The oxygen remains in your bloodstream and the benefits can stay with you for weeks afterwards.

Clean up your liver

Your liver is a master recycler – a rubbish collector extraordinaire. It receives all the substances – nutrients, toxins, and medications – that are processed by your body's various systems dividing them into 'good' and 'bad'. The 'bad' are redirected to the appropriate elimination channels to be expelled, and the 'good' – mainly amino acids, proteins and fats – are broken down for storage and conversion into energy for the cells.

Over time, and particularly if you smoke, drink too much and/ or eat processed, unhealthy foods, your liver can become overwhelmed and stop functioning as efficiently as it used to. As it struggles to cope with the toxic overload, poisons build up in your blood. This can affect your brain, reducing function and ultimately permanently damaging it. Apart from the obvious – stopping smoking and drinking altogether, and eating well – there are effective ways to assist your liver in its clean up.

Action plan

- **Take milk thistle capsules** This is a herbal remedy known to help liver and gall bladder problems. You can buy them in most health food shops.

- **Eat garlic in natural or capsule form** Garlic triggers the production of enzymes in your liver, which protect and help detox it.

- **Try dandelion root supplements** These stimulate bile production, and it is bile that removes toxins from the liver, leaving it clear to continue 'rubbish collecting'.

- **Give yourself an enema** This is an excellent way to detox the liver as it quickly accesses the hepatic vein, which lies just inside the large intestine, and carries the detox to the liver within a matter of seconds. Gerson therapy advocates coffee enemas, to shock the liver into dumping its toxins and releasing bile. A wheatgrass enema has a similar effect, but as it is packed with vitamins, enzymes, beta-carotene and chlorophyll, it also re-energises and oxygenates the liver, giving your immune system a thorough reboot in the process. You can do these at home as the tube only goes 4cm (1 $\frac{1}{2}$in) into your rectum, so there is no risk of perforation. You can buy an enema bag and large bottle of distilled water from your local chemist and research how to do it on the internet. Detox Enema Coffee is available on Amazon from the Organic Coffee Cleanse Company.

Boost your kidneys

You have two kidneys and they are responsible for removing acidic waste from your body via your urine. They are your body's alkalinity watchdogs – the more acidic the environment in your body, the greater the opportunity for chronic disease. Your kidneys need large quantities of water to flush everything through every day. Without adequate hydration, they slow down and stop functioning properly, and eventually, gallstones may develop. Dehydration also slows your brain. As mentioned already, your brain is 73 per cent water and loss of fluid equal to two per cent of your body weight has been shown to affect decision-making[4] and creates problems with focus, cognitive and motor skills, and memory as your brain literally shrinks in size.[5] Dehydration adversely affects your memory and clarity of thinking in much the same way as being drunk.

Action plan

- **Increase your water intake** Put a jug of (filtered) water on your desk or kitchen table and down a glass or two every hour. As your brain is three-quarters water, the more often water flushes through your system, the more toxins are excreted via your urine and the sharper your brain becomes.

- **Swap your coffee for a kidney-boosting herbal tea or juice** Dandelion or nettle tea flush out uric acid. Ginger and turmeric added to a cup of hot water will also help remove excess minerals and salts. Fresh, organic cranberry or grape juice also flushes out uric acid.

Help your lymphatic and glymphatic systems

The lymphatic system is a complex network that, rather like the blood vessels, runs throughout your entire body, lying just below the surface of the skin. There are two main parts: the lymph vessels, which carry lymph fluid, and lymph nodes. Lymph is a clear watery liquid that carries cell waste to the other elimination organs for disposal and protects you from all the bacteria, viruses and toxins it meets along the way. The lymph nodes are the tiny kidney-shaped nodules found in your neck, armpits, chest, stomach, pelvis and groin, which act as gatekeepers, filtering and preventing invasion by bacteria, viruses and other dangerous intruders that could cause serious illness.

Up to now the lymphatic system has been thought of as a system that runs only from the neck downwards, but recent research has categorically proven that another system, the glymphatic system, extends up and around your head in the dura, the leathery outer coating of the brain. The glymph system connects with the lymph system at the neck and is named after the glial cells that play a fundamental part in the process; glial cells feed the brain's neurons, and protect them from damage.

The glymphatic system, the brain's rubbish collector, runs in parallel to the arteries and as they expand and contract it acts like a toxin-drainage system, removing waste products and efficiently dealing with any build-up of fluid that might be harmful to the brain. The glial cells – the astroglia specifically – pump cerebrospinal fluid (CSF) into and around the brain and spinal cord, clearing proteins from the interstitial space between them while you sleep. Latest studies seem to show that problems with flow in the glymphatic system may correlate with the start and progression of neurological issues. Type 2 diabetes has been shown to slow CSF clearing by a factor of three.[6]

The glymphatic system becomes less efficient with age and recent research shows that disrupted sleep patterns also slows down glymphatic flow and so toxin removal, allowing disruption that may be connected with the development of Parkinson's disease. Stiffening of the blood vessels due to high blood pressure can also reduce its capacity to clean up toxins in the brain as it's the pulsating arterial walls that drives its flow.

Action plan

- **Move about more** Lymph needs to be moved to work effectively. Increasing your heart rate, particularly with exercise that jars your skeletal system a little (such as jogging or bouncing on a rebounder) will help to get your lymph moving. Exercise also reduces high blood pressure and arterial stiffness; aerobic exercise can reverse problems with glymph flow.[7]

- **Reverse your gravity** Learn some yoga head stands or shoulder stands, as this can get your lymph/glymph flowing – or invest in an inversion table (see Chapter 11).

- **Have a massage** An effective lymph massage can dissolve blockages in the nodes over a period of time.

- **Take herbal remedies** Both red clover and goose grass stimulate and drain the glymphatic/lymphatic system, reducing inflammation in the process. Apex Energetics produces Lymph-Max that can stimulate lymphatic flow.

- **Try dry skin brushing** Give your skin a quick scrub with a long-handled brush each morning before you shower. This will rid it of the toxins you sweated out each night and stimulate your lymph and blood circulation.

● **Take nitric-oxide supplements** These have been shown to strengthen lymphatic contraction and reduce arterial stiffness, which reduces inflammation in the brain, boosting cognitive function.

● **Sleep for longer** The glymphatic system is most active at night when you are asleep. Research carried out on mice shows that the volume of interstitial space increases by 60 per cent at that time and that exchange of CSF and interstitial fluid also increases, which speeds up the removal of amyloid and other neurotoxic waste products accumulated during daylight. Broken sleep patterns are now thought to be linked to the development of Parkinson's disease.[8]

● **Book an Indian head massage** A massage that focuses on your face, scalp, neck and ears boosts blood flow and glymphatic circulation in your head, so optimising waste clearance from the brain cells while you sleep at night. According to brain scans, lying flat while you have a massage, rather than sitting, is the most effective way of mobilising the glymphatic system.[9]

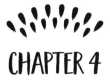

CHAPTER 4

THE HIDDEN ENEMIES

*'There are more viruses on Earth than stars
in the universe.'*

CARL ZIMMER, JOURNALIST AND AUTHOR

You are probably well aware of the obvious physical influences on brain function, such as what you eat, the exercise you take, and the realities of your daily routine, work, and home life. However, there are a number of invisible factors you may not have considered. A wide range of common viruses, parasites, fungi and bacteria are known to influence the brain, and the effects may linger long after any initial signs have disappeared (not all will have obvious symptoms). Mould is rarely thought of in relation to brain issues, yet it is one of the most dangerous neurotoxins known to man.

Considering the impact of each of these hidden enemies in turn is a worthwhile exercise for anyone wanting to improve their brain function. And I offer advice on what you can do to eliminate each aggressor from your system, thereby reducing the toxic load on your brain.

Viruses

Infectious agents that only replicate inside the living cells of an organism, viruses come in many shapes and sizes. Some are spread through the air, for example, when people cough or sneeze. Others move via contaminated foods, dirty hands or polluted water. Yet more are carried by insects and can be transferred by bites or travel in bodily fluids. There are around 500 hundred viruses known to affect the brain, many at a subtle level.[1] Much of the time they are contained by the immune system and don't become neuroinvasive, but some are more aggressive. These may lie dormant within your body, hiding in a biofilm designed to avoid detection by your immune system. At times of stress, when your immunity is low, they often re-emerge, triggering a host of symptoms. If you are struggling with cognitive problems, memory issues and brain fog, then it may be worth considering whether one or more viruses may be at the root of your difficulties.

Invisible, long-term viral warfare

Viruses can cross the blood–brain barrier in a number of ways, avoiding ordinary means of immune-detection. They enter your central nervous system (CNS) – the spinal cord and brain – via the nerves of your peripheral nervous system. They can penetrate your neurons, travelling via the axons to the brain.

The hardest-hitting viruses can cause serious damage to the brain – but it can depend on the age of the individual under attack and the type of virus. The Coxsackie virus can trigger meningitis, inflammation of the spinal cord and the brain. Cytomegalovirus, rubella, and lymphocytic choriomeningitis virus can cause hydrocephalus (swelling due to an accumulation of cerebrospinal fluid in the brain) and have been shown to reduce mental function and IQ. West Nile virus is responsible for neurological problems in the elderly, whereas at the other end of the age scale, cytomegalovirus can cause permanent brain damage in the foetus and young still developing brain, but does no harm to a fully developed brain.[2]

Different viruses affect different parts of the brain too. I have covered some of the common culprits below. The herpes simplex virus, for example, targets the temporal lobes, whereas West Nile virus attacks the cerebral cortex. Initially untraceable viral attacks can cause neurological problems decades later, too. The aptly named Wild type vesicular stomatitis virus (VSV) reduces the numbers of serotonin neurons in the brain, leaving its host with life-long depression long after it has been removed by the immune system. With no residual evidence of its invisible sabotage there are no clues for either patient or doctor when mental health issues arise that might point the way towards successful treatment.[3]

Human papilloma virus (HPV)

The human papilloma virus (HPV), best known as the cause of cervical cancer, can have a major impact on the brain. There are more than 170 different viruses in the HPV 'family', and while some trigger lower-level symptoms such as benign lesions, genital warts and facial palsy, others are responsible for more serious brain-related illnesses, including head and neck cancer. HPV symptoms often trigger anxiety and depression, and excessive stress, drinking and smoking are thought to block the body's capacity to rid itself of the virus.

Read up on the latest research about the widely pushed HPV vaccines, and the importance of taking responsibility for managing your own health becomes clear. The vaccines have never been proven to prevent cervical or any other cancer yet, evidence shows that certain ingredients in the vaccines may have serious side effects. Participants in the trials reported developing new medical conditions including neurological syndromes and autoimmune disorders. People have also reported headaches, fatigue, cognitive dysfunction, interrupted sleep, blurring of vision, neuropathic pain, and motor symptoms.[4]

Most adults have been exposed to HPV at some point, so women should not miss out on an annual smear test. HPV is usually transmitted through sexual or skin-to-skin contact and 90 per cent of infections clear up on their own. Catch the problem early and the virus never need develop into something more serious. But if it does, the latest research shows that BioBran, made from the husks of rice broken down by shitake mushrooms, is effective at both preventing and eliminating HPV from the system.[5] With no side effects, a pill a day sounds a less immune compromising solution than many pharmaceutical options. www.healthy.co.uk.

Human herpes viruses (HHV)

Only nine out of the 130 identified herpes viruses are known to affect human beings, known as Human herpes viruses or HHVs. Of those nine, six can damage your brain – HHV-3 (varicella zoster virus, VZV), HHV-4 (Epstein-Barr virus, EBV), HHV-5 (Human cytomegalovirus), HHV-6A and HHV-6B (Human herpes virus 6A and B), HHV-7 (Human herpes virus 7) and finally, HHV-8 (Kaposi's sarcoma-associated herpes virus, mainly found in those affected by HIV).

Recent research described in the journal *Neuron* carried out autopsies on 622 people who died with Alzheimer's in their brains. They found a clear connection between the virus and the Alzheimer's and identified two strains of the herpes virus – HHV-6A and HHV-7 – in one third of the brains.[6]

The main HHV culprits

The word herpes comes from the Greek *'herpein'* meaning 'to creep' – underlining its ability to do exactly that, accessing your brain and spinal column via your nerves.[7]

HHV-3 Varicella zoster virus (VZV) – the chickenpox virus
This is one of the more common herpes viruses and it is accepted as a fact of life that once you've had it (usually in childhood), the virus lies dormant in your system and can be 'reactivated' in adulthood as shingles. Recent Swedish research indicates that there may be a link between this virus, particularly in its adult form, and long-term memory and cognitive impairments as a result of neuronal damage resulting from infection with VZV. The virus was also found in the spinal fluid of a group of 72 patients suffering from stroke, encephalitis and a range of other brain infections.[8]

HHV-4 Epstein-Barr virus This widespread virus causes glandular fever, and is an example of the type of herpes that most of us carry without being aware we have it. It too can cause a range of brain-related symptoms. These tend to present more in those whose immune systems are already compromised as a result of chronic trauma and at times of stress, it can 'flare up', even if it has been dormant for many years. Latest reports suggest that Epstein-Barr may be a trigger for both Lyme disease and shingles and that there may be a connection with multiple sclerosis.[9]

HHV-5 Human cytomegalovirus (HCMV) Widely present in the general population, HCMV is another virus that remains dormant in your body, re-emerging at times of high stress and immune-system depletion. According to US

continued...

researchers, 58.9 per cent of people aged 6 and older are infected with it and a whopping 90.8 per cent over the age of 80 will test positive.[10]

Congenital HCMV is the leading infectious cause of deafness, low IQ and learning difficulties in children[11]. About 5 per cent of babies that are born infected with HCMV (5 in every 1,000 live births) will go on to develop cerebral calcification that triggers dramatic decreasing of IQ levels, psychomotor retardation and sensorineural deafness. Cognitive issues also affect babies infected after birth, who develop brain problems later in life.[12]

HHV-6 and HHV-7 Research now shows that both viruses are linked to low-grade inflammation of the brain. In some cases, HHV-6 can cause cognitive dysfunction and may be a trigger for both multiple sclerosis and chronic fatigue syndrome. High levels have been found in the brain biopsies of patients with epilepsy suggesting it may play a role in causing seizures. It is estimated that 90 per cent of the US population over the age of 5 have had HHV-6 or HHV-7, despite the majority showing no obvious symptoms.[13]

HHV-6A and HHV-6B are two more recently identified, closely related variants of the HHV-6 virus, associated with encephalitis, meningitis and brain inflammation[14]. But because HHV-6A is not yet detectable from a blood test it is difficult to estimate what per centage of people with HHV-6 have this additional variation, but it highlights once more how vital it is for brain health to treat for the possibility of invasion by the herpes virus.

A recent study has also found that HHV-6 and HHV-7 viruses are likely to be implicated in longer term development of

continued...

Alzheimer's.[15] Initial findings seem to indicate that they continually emit low levels of proteins, which interact with genes known to play a role in Alzheimer's disease. When they start actively reproducing, they appear to speed up the Alzheimer's-related protein build-up that ultimately leads to system failure for the brain.

HIV (human immunodeficiency virus)

HIV is another example of a virus that many people live with for years before becoming symptomatic, but even in its earliest stages, before any obvious symptoms appear, it impacts on the brain. In 2016, the UK government estimated that around 13,500 people in the country were living with undiagnosed HIV.[16] This could mean that the virus is affecting their brains without them being aware of it. A 2017 study by researchers at Stellenbosch University, South Africa, used functional magnetic resonance imaging (fMRI) to observe the brains of HIV-positive subjects undertaking specific tasks. They saw that in the HIV-positive group, there was reduced blood flow to the striatal region, which relates to higher motor functions. They also observed reduced blood flow to the nucleus accumbens – the part of the forebrain where reduced blood flow has been linked to apathy.

Turning the tables: Using harmful viruses to heal

It's not all bad news on the virus front. Conventional medicine has begun to use the adaptive skills of viruses for the successful treatment of brain cancer. Varicella zoster, myxoma and other herpes viruses are being used to target, infect and kill glioblastomas in adults[17] and a genetically modified version of the herpes virus has been used successfully, with no side effects, on children with glioblastomas.[18]

Recently, researchers from Duke University, USA, used a genetically modified polio virus to extend survival rates in adults with brain cancer. It not only destroyed their tumours, but also triggered an immune response that reactivated the patient's immune systems against glioblastoma herpes.[19]

Action plan

So how do you destroy viruses that may be affecting your brain? Conventional medicine has little in its toolbox of pharmaceutical options to fight brain-weakening viruses and they are rarely on the radar of a medical treatment plan. Antibiotics simply don't work and your doctor is likely to advise you to go home and wait for any symptoms to pass. is A vital first step on the road back to brain health is to become aware that viruses are potential antagonists. There are steps you can take to boost your immune response and antiviral capacity.

➤ **Consult a naturopath, a NAET (nambridripad allergy elimination technique) practitioner, or kinesiologist** They can run assessments to determine which specific virus may be affecting you.

- **Boost your vitamin D levels** Keep your vitamin D levels high and your immune system should be able to fight off most viruses – the main source of the vitamin is sunlight. Ask your doctor for a blood test. A level of 60 is optimal, but if you find yourself in a lower range it can be boosted intravenously or you can take a daily supplement of 10,000iu until your numbers rise. (See Chapter 7 for more on vitamin D.)

- **Look into natural remedies** These can be fast-acting and more effective at wiping out viruses than the antiviral drugs your doctor might prescribe. If you take action as soon as you are diagnosed with a viral infection you can prevent damage or inflammation in your brain. A combination of colloidal silver, tea tree oil, apple cider vinegar and mushroom tincture packs a powerful punch – see www.Reboothealth. co.uk/shingles.

- **Increase your enzyme intake** Eat three portions of either pineapple and/or mango daily – both contain proteolytic enzymes that strip away the protective outer layers and heads of viruses. A German study found these enzymes to be as effective as some standard antiviral medications at relieving the pain from shingles and healing the rash.[20]

- **Chew liquorice root** Liquorice contains two potent antivirals, the triterpenes GL and GA. You can also buy liquorice tincture from a herbalist, or capsules from a health store; check the labels though as you should not buy DGL (deglycyrrhizinated) liquorice root as the active ingredient has been removed[21].

- **Take oregano** Add fresh or dried oregano to your cooking, or take the oil (capsules or concentrate) as it's one of the most potent natural antivirals and immune-boosting remedies.

- **Take elderberry syrup** Viruses clad themselves in sharp spikes, to protect themselves and to attack and overrun your healthy cells. Research has shown that protective compounds in elderberries wipe out those spikes in a couple of days, preventing any further spreading of the virus – hence its nickname the 'virus terminator'. An Israeli study, looking at viruses and the efficacy of elderberry syrup, showed that those who took a daily dose recovered far more quickly than the control group – 20 per cent were better within 24 hours, 70 per cent in 48 hours, and 90 per cent had recovered completely in three days.[22]

- **Use colloidal silver** – but never for more than 14 days at a time. Dr Martin Hum, of the Institute for Optimum Nutrition, London, lists colloidal silver as one of the fastest-acting natural antiviral remedies. Use in spray or drop form (you can spray your throat, nose and even infected eyes) for short periods when needed. Make sure you buy true colloidal silver, rather than ionic or silver-protein alternatives, which are not as powerful. Effective against HIV, herpes, hepatitis C and shingles, colloidal silver works by suffocating the viruses. Colloidal silver can also be used for bacterial infections (see page 74).

Parasitic infections

You are more likely to be subject to infection from parasites when your immune system is weak. And people are particularly vulnerable whilst undergoing treatment for cancer, or long-term, or chronic conditions such as HIV.

The parasites may initially colonise the gut, but they can also travel to your brain, where they may protect themselves from discovery by the immune system by hiding themselves away in tiny cysts that even antibiotics can't break down. Pets, particularly dogs and cats, may play host to highly contagious roundworms that can migrate to humans and move upwards from their intestines to infect eyes and the brain.

Toxoplasmosis

Toxoplasma gondii is one of the few parasites that can cross the blood–brain barrier and damage the spinal cord and brain. Between 30 and 50 per cent of the population may be infected with it and it is most commonly picked up by eating undercooked meat, a fact that isn't widely known, as we tend to think of it as a parasite spread only in·cat poo. A healthy immune system will keep the parasite in check, but in individuals whose immunity is suppressed, it can cause a range of problems in the brain such as inflammation, abscesses, headaches, seizures, confusion and even loss of consciousness in some instances. If the parasite takes hold in the eye, Toxoplasmosis can destroy the retina, damaging the brain and cause mental disturbances.

Fascinatingly, researchers recently linked colonisation by the parasite with a significant elevation in risk-taking behaviour, indicating it may have an impact on personality, suggesting that it invades the frontal cortex. If you have been infected, you will have antibodies for life,[23] but recent research shows that you may also have the parasite for life and the infection can flare up again in times of stress and immune system suppression, but a healthy immune system will prevent re-activation. For most people the symptoms will clear up within a few weeks or months. The main risk is to contract toxoplasmosis in pregnancy, as it can potentially affect an unborn child, resulting in a smaller or larger head than normal, and possible learning difficulties, seizures, and loss of vision.

Malaria

Transmitted through the bite of an infected mosquito, malaria has killed millions of people around the globe. The malarial danger zone is centred in Africa, but carrier mosquitos are found across Asia, and in Central and South America, and anyone in these regions risks infection if bitten by one. Cerebral malaria, where the parasite invades the brain tissue, leads to loss of consciousness and death if it is not treated immediately. With medical treatment, there is still a 15–20 per cent risk of mortality and you can be left with serious cognitive issues.

Bilharzia

Also known as schistosomiasis, this results from infection by parasitic flatworms, or flukes. Roughly 240 million people are infected each year in tropical and sub-tropical countries, and although it is usually associated with liver, kidney and bladder problems, the parasites can later invade the brain causing serious issues. Many infected people show no symptoms. The parasites are often picked up through swimming in infected lakes and other fresh water sources. The larvae break through the skin, then travel via the blood, to lodge in the organs, and later move into the spinal cord and up to the brain, causing swelling, seizures and epilepsy.

Giardiasis

This infection is caused by a microscopic parasite called giardia lamblia. Picked up from contact with unwashed surfaces, faecal matter, uncooked foods, contaminated water or simply from another infected person, giardiasis has long been connected to intestinal problems, particularly severe diarrhoea, bloating and abdominal pain. Recent research, however, indicates that giardiasis may lead to inflammation of the brain and more serious complications, particularly if contracted by young children.[24] Long-term diarrhoea during early childhood has been found to affect visual–motor coordination, short-term auditory memory, information processing, and cortical cognitive function.[25] The nutritional deficiencies caused by the severe diarrhoea – particularly of vitamin B12, and minerals such as zinc, and iron – also contribute to poor cognitive and language developmental skills.

Action plan

Parasite infestation can be prevented, see below, but there are also a number of remedies that can help if you have been infected.

- **Wash your hands frequently throughout the day** Always wash them before eating, and after using the bathroom. It is especially important to wash your hands after contact with pets.

- **Wash all fruits and vegetables** It is important to wash them thoroughly before you eat them, whether you are eating them raw or cooked. Read the advice on organic food in chapter 7 for more on how to minimise your pesticide consumption.

- **Cook meat thoroughly** Raw meat can harbour parasites.

- **Do a regular parasite cleanse of your home** Whether you have symptoms or not, it is sensible to do a parasite cleanse once or twice a year. Your local health store will offer a variety of options or visit a herbalist or nutritionist for advice.

Useful remedies

Artemisinin and artemether Research has shown the antimalarial compound artemisinin to be one of the most effective natural remedies for toxoplasmosis.[26] In tests a derivative of artemisinin, artemether, was ten times more effective against the parasite.[27] Consult your doctor for dosage.

Nutmeg Research indicates that nutmeg oil is effective against parasites and bacteria. It can also enhance memory and reduce depression.[28]

Powder of mimosa pudica This is an Ayurvedic remedy for cleansing the body of parasites. Take $\frac{1}{2}$ teaspoon of the powder twice a day for 3 months, or drink it as a tea.

Take berberine Research published in 2012 found that berberine, an alkaloid found in goldenseal, destroys the parasite that causes toxoplasmosis.[29] The usual dose is 900–2,000mg a day, divided into three to four doses. Take before or with a meal.

Invest in a Hulda Clark zapper This is a small, inexpensive frequency machine that destroys parasites simply and non-invasively. If you search for this on the Internet, you will find disparaging comments sitting alongside equally enthusiastic reviews. I was introduced to this machine 40 years ago when travelling around India. A test in a holistic clinic showed that there were wriggling parasites clearly visible in my blood. I used the zapper for 10 minutes, twice a day, and four days later there was no sign of the wrigglers; I have been a convert ever since.

Bacteria

Fewer than one per cent of bacteria are harmful to the body, but some of these are particularly damaging to the brain. In meningitis, for example, the cocci bacteria can cause the membrane around the brain and the spinal cord (meninges) to swell, which may result in permanent brain damage and loss of function. MRSA (methicillin-resistant staphylococcus aureus), the antibiotic-resistant 'super bug', can also lead to meningitis and pneumonia.

I'll describe the gut-brain axis and the impact of the gut microbiome on brain function and health in more detail in Chapter 8, but I wanted to mention some new research that complicates our existing understanding of the bacteria–brain connection and provides evidence that there are bacteria in the brain itself. In 2018, scientists announced that they had made an unexpected and fascinating discovery. Where once the brain had been thought of as a 'sterile site', researchers involved in a study looking at the differences in the brains of schizophrenic and healthy subjects, observed significant concentrations of bacteria in both. Bacteria were found in several different parts of the brain, and a large quantity in the astrocytes, the star-shaped brain cells found close to the blood–brain barrier. When the researchers sequenced genetic material from the bacteria, they found that most of the microbes were from groups that are typically found in the human gut. In a subsequent study, the same team found that mice, too, have brains teeming with bacteria, and that when laboratory mice are engineered to be 'bacteria-free', their brains are correspondingly sterile. The precise role of all these bacteria is unclear, but it is interesting that, just as the gut behaves in some ways like a 'second brain' (see page 173), so too perhaps the brain has its own microbiome. More research is needed to explore this connection, so watch this space!

Action plan

- **Minimise exposure to bacteria** This can be difficult as they are everywhere – so wash your hands frequently throughout the day, particularly before eating, or after bumping into someone coughing, sneezing or blowing their nose. Become aware of how often you touch your eyes, nose or mouth. Touch a door handle, or hold on to a rail in the bus or train, and then rub your nose or touch your lips and your chance of infection multiplies.

- **Use colloidal silver** It can be used as a spray, cream for the skin, or as a gel dressings for wounds, but never for longer than 14 days at a time. Colloidal silver has been scientifically proven to destroy bacteria that are resistant to the strongest antibiotics. In the 1980s, at UCLA medical school, Larry C. Ford MD documented over 650 different disease-causing pathogens that were destroyed in minutes when exposed to small amounts. In addition, a study published in the *Journal of Alternative and Complementary Medicine* supported ionic colloidal silver as a broad-spectrum antimicrobial agent against both aerobic and anaerobic bacteria. Make sure you buy true colloidal silver, rather than ionic or silver-protein alternatives, which are not as powerful.

- **Take berberine** This is an alkaloid found in goldenseal that has been shown to be effective against MRSA and other bacteria. The usual dose is 900–2,000mg a day, divided into three to four doses; take it before or with a meal.

- **Take oregano oil** Take two or three capsules every four hours and the symptoms of bacterial-based food poisoning disappear in 24 hours – much faster than the antibiotics your doctor may recommend.

- **Take probiotics** A high level of 'good' bacteria in your gut will reduce the effects of any 'bad' bacteria. Symprove sell a 12-week programme of multi-strain, live and active bacteria, that includes *E. faecium, L. rhamnosus, L. acidophilus and L. plantarum.* Research shows that for a bacteria-based product to make it through your stomach unharmed by your digestive acids it has to 'survive, arrive and thrive'. Symprove was the only product that managed 100 per cent of all three in a study carried out by the University of London. www.symprove.com

Mould

Mould is a fungus that can undermine your brain in myriad ways. It is not on the average doctor's list of possible triggers for illness and it doesn't show up in blood tests. Very few people think of it as a threat, yet it is one of the most dangerous toxins. According to World Health Organisation estimates, dampness and mould affect 10–50 per cent of homes in Europe, North America, Australia, India and Japan.[30] And in the US, the figure is even higher, at approximately 50–80 per cent.[31] Anybody living in an old, damp house, in a damp climate will have high levels of mould in their surroundings.

There are thousands of mould variations. Most are harmless, but it's black mould, a toxic variety, that causes the majority of health problems. Some mould is obvious, for example, as mould spots around the edges of baths and sinks or visible damp patches, but much of it isn't as it's under the floors, behind water-using appliances, kitchen units or wallpaper, under your carpet or behind your old kitchen units. Damp, lack of light and air, and 'food' (for example, plasterboard, dust, wood – basically anything that contains cellulose) provide the ideal conditions for mould to not only survive, but multiply. If you remove just one of those factors, mould can't continue to grow.

Mould toxins are made up of fatty acid molecules and they are deposited wherever there is fat – and the brain is 60 per cent fat. For the 25 per cent of the population who have a genetic predisposition that prevents them from effectively clearing biotoxins, mould can be toxic for the brain. These people have the HLA-DRBQ gene and don't produce the antibodies needed to defend against and eradicate mould toxins, but store them instead. There is not much recent research on the genetic connection, but the jury is no longer out – mould can be dangerous for our brains, triggering chronic low-level inflammation and reducing mental function.

How does mould affect the brain?

Breathing in mould spores from the air, or eating too much mould-friendly food, raises the levels of candida and other moulds in your body to such an extent that your immune system struggles to protect you. Candida is a common fungus that can give you similar symptoms to a nervous breakdown or depression and may be the trigger behind a diagnosis of meningitis.[32] (See also Candida: The dangers of internal mould, page 79–80.) In studies on mice, mould exposure was found to impact negatively on memory recall and to increase the symptoms of anxiety.[33] It has been found to affect children's brains too – a Polish study looking at children's IQ found that those who had lived the longest in a home with visible mould spores saw the most significant reduction in their IQ.

Mould is poisonous to brain cells. In a recent study, SPECT brain scans (a type of nuclear imaging that helps create a 3D picture of the brain) were carried out after participants had been exposed to mould. The results showed staggering degrees of abnormality in different areas of the brain: 67.7 per cent had areas in their temporal lobes, 61.3 per cent in the frontal lobes, 45.2 per cent in the basal ganglia, 29 per cent in the thalamus, and 12.9 per cent in their parietal lobes.[34] Mould can cause mood swings and switch your brain into a state of rage, anger or irritation. An overgrowth in the brain can overwhelm you with sadness and depression and anxiety, and affect the clarity of your thinking, including your contextual and spatial memory.[35] Research also shows that mould inhalation correlates with decreased neurogenesis, and an increase in inflammation. Mould also loves damp and warmth, so the vitreous liquid in the eye is another perfect place for it to lodge. Clear up any mould there and your eyesight may well improve, too.[36]

Don't confuse mould allergy and mould toxicity

Mould allergy, a reaction to inhaling the spores, and mould toxicity poisoning are two separate complaints. The first causes fever-like symptoms and mimics the common allergic-style response seen in hay fever, for example, itching, constant tiredness, eye and throat irritation and headaches. In contrast, mould-toxicity poisoning is far harder to diagnose and often triggers symptoms that are easily misdiagnosed as neurological and auto-immune disorders, from fibromyalgia to chronic fatigue syndrome (CFS). Neurotoxic poisoning from mould can cause irreversible nervous system damage, killing off brain cells and permanently altering cell structure and receptor sensitivity. Symptoms may show themselves as headaches, dizziness, seizures, movement disorders, cranial nerve issues or neuromuscular problems, with declining levels of reaction time, cognition, verbal learning, recall, concentration and balance.[37]

Action plan

• **Check your home and office for mould** Look behind sinks, showers and appliances, and underneath your skirting, floorboards or behind any walls made from plasterboard – its cellulose-rich composition makes it mould's favourite feeding ground. If you find mould, send samples to a lab for analysis. Try Emlab.com, they can run an ERMI (environmental relative mouldiness index) test, which analyses the dust in your home to identify the quantity and different types of the moulds present – it identifies up to 36 species.

• **Rent a de-humidifier** This will remove excess water from the atmosphere. Consider buying an air purifier, too.

• **Clean the mould off the walls and surfaces** Wear a good-quality mask while you do this to ensure you inhale as little as possible. Try natural non-toxic anti-mould formulas: hydrogen peroxide, grapefruit seed extract, neat vinegar and tea tree oil are all powerful natural fungicides. In severe cases, you will need to call in an expert to treat it.

• **Check if you suffer from mould sensitivity** If you are affected by mould, your contrast vision may be reduced as the mould affects the nerve cells. Ken Hudnall from the environmental agency of the USA developed an online visual contrast sensitivity (VCS) test that can be done for a small charge. Further monitoring with the test will tell you when you are clear of the infection. www.vcstest.com

• **Sign up for a few sessions in a pressurised hyperbaric chamber** This can help can lift the 'fog' – research shows it takes around 20 sessions to clear the fungus.

- **Take caprylic acid** A saturated fatty acid found in coconut and palm oils, caprylic acid essentially makes tiny holes in the cell walls of any invading yeast, killing them in the process.

- **Take artichoke leaf extract** A study published in the Journal of Agricultural Food Chemistry in 2004 found that taking extract of artichoke leaf successfully destroyed moulds and yeasts.

- **Install a diffuser and experiment with essential oils** Try 2 or 3 drops of Myrrh as it's an anti-microbial, anti-fungal, and anti-inflammatory that can also raise your body's resistance to mould. Or fill a diffuser with Young Living's thieves oil, which is a combination of clove, cinnamon, rosemary, eucalyptus, and lemon. This oil works by surrounding the mould, and literally eating the spores. Thyme, clove, sage and cinnamon essential oils are also effective.

- **Download my e-book:** *The Mould Menace:Fix your Body, Fix your Brain* from Amazon, for a comprehensive overview of all the issues.

Candida – The dangers of internal mould

Candida albicans is a yeast that lives in the small intestine and colon. We all have it in our bodies and it is supposed to be there, alongside the yeasts, bacteria and viruses that live in the gut – and it is estimated that around 70 per cent of us have it in elevated levels, usually in our small and large intestines. However, less well known is the fact that candida can spread from these areas throughout your whole body, moving its threadlike roots to burrow its way right up to your brain. New research shows that candida can cause memory problems and brain abnormalities similar to those of Alzheimer's Disease.[38] The fungus enters your brain, penetrating the blood–brain

continued...

barrier and affects the brain's immune cells, triggering an inflammatory response and forming structures in the brain similar to amyloid plaques. Research compared mice with candida to mice without and found that those who had candida showed reduced spatial memory. When the infection cleared, their spatial memory went back to normal. It is possible that fungi may similarly be involved in the development of chronic neurodegenerative conditions like Parkinson's disease and multiple sclerosis. In time science will tell us.[39]

What you can do to help

Cut out candida-loving foods and those you are sensitive to Usually they are one and the same. Try to cut out anything with sugar in it, along with alcohol, mushrooms, cheese, bread, fruit and fruit juice.

Take caprylic acid Found in coconut and palm oil, this fatty acid is an essential in the fight against the fungi. It is absorbed by your intestinal walls and kills both the yeast form of candida and the more invasive mycelial threads, without harming your good gut bacteria.

Take goldenseal This is a powerful anti-fungal that not only kills bacteria, viruses and parasites, but also stops the virulent die-off that you can experience when candida dies, as this releases large quantities of toxins.

Try a wheatgrass enema implant Wheatgrass contains natural chemicals that rapidly kill the yeast.

Take more probiotics Make sure you up your dose of probiotics in order to repopulate your gut – high doses of Lactobacillus acidophilus dds1 and Bifidobacterium bifidum are effective.

Take oregano oil Four drops daily in a glass of water wipes out any yeast in its vicinity.[40]

Electromagnetic fields

We are surrounded by invisible, inaudible electromagnetic frequencies, or EMFs, and are bombarded daily by innumerable rays. Everything from your Wi-Fi router, phone, tablet, or computer to the televisions and electronic radios, dishwashers, microwaves, ovens and washing machines that sit continually 'on', gently emanate a frequency of their own and add to the mix. And it is not just in your home or office. If you live in a city, you will be affected by the strength of the waves emanating from your neighbours' houses too. It's no better in the countryside. The electricity station down the road and the pylons that cross the woods and fields are all invisibly pulsating frequencies that are usually, to differing degrees, incompatible with human health.

Your brain, mobile phones and the arrival of 5G

And last, but certainly not least, a very 21st-century assailant, 5G, or the Fifth Generation of mobile phone technology, whose invisible effects on our brains will not be clear for some time – although all indications are that this will be one enemy it will be extremely hard to beat. This technology uses frequencies that are less crowded than the existing systems and allows you to download at a speed of over 1,000Mbit/s (1Gbit/s), more than 100 times faster than the current UK 4G network. It can handle a far wider range of the new technologies – for example, driverless cars, manufacturing sensors and more connected home devices.

In the UK, the 5G roll-out plan involves installing short masts (rather than the tall mobile phone towers we see now) that will broadcast their radio waves as widely as possible across the country. The spread is far greater than ever before. Masts will be sited on telegraph poles and street lamps, in parks, and on the roof tops of schools, and government-owned buildings. And the available science clearly indicates that their frequencies will have a detrimental effect on the brain. Never before will the human race have been bombarded by electromagnetic frequencies of such high levels. More than 240 scientists have now appealed to the United Nations to reduce public exposure to 5G rather than increase it. They are calling for a moratorium on 5G concluding that, 'RF-EMF has been proven to be harmful for humans and the environment'.[41]

Cell-phone brain drain

The cancer epidemiology update, a comprehensive review of radiofrequency EMF fields and their effects on humans and animals, concludes that scientific evidence shows radiofrequency radiation is carcinogenic to humans.[42] Most studies of mobile phones and brain cancer have only looked at cases where a person has used a cell phones for five years or less. However, serious studies that have examined people who have used cell phones for 10 years or more, have found a 50–80 per cent increased risk of brain cancer.[43] They have also found direct connections with damage to the brain and the nervous system, as well as sleep patterns, and fertility levels.[44] A 2019 study of students in schools sited near cell phone towers found that their exposure to higher radio frequency levels was associated with impacts on motor skills, memory and attention.[45] Examples of other effects linked to phone masts in research studies include neuropsychiatric problems, diabetes, headaches, sleep problems and genetic damage. A 2010 landmark review looked at 56 studies and found that, even at very low intensities, frequencies impacted on reproduction, permeability of the blood–brain barrier, behaviour, cellular and metabolic behaviour and showed an increased cancer risk.[46] Martin L. Pall, Professor Emeritus of Biochemistry and Basic Medical Sciences at Washington State University, USA, has said that mobile phones attack our nervous systems, including our brains, leading to widespread neurological and neuropsychiatric effects. The Israeli, Finnish and French governments have all issued 5G health warnings. As yet the British government has not.

Action plan

● **Check the radio frequencies of places where you spend most time** I like the inexpensive Gauss meter; you can get them online.

● **Swap from wireless to wired where possible** Put the wire back into your computer, keyboard, mouse and printers. Check your existing router, and replace it if necessary with a low EMF model. Fixed house phones are perfectly safe.

● **Invest in air-tube headphones** Ditch the blue-tooth. Air-tube headphones reduce the EMF radiation from your cell phone.

● **Replace all 'smart' home devices** This includes your power meters as well as the TV and other devices.

● **Make your bedroom an EMF-free zone** For example, turn your electric switches and sockets off when you go to bed, and remove any electronic clock-radio from your bedside table. Don't sleep next to a switched on mobile phone and switch off any plugs directly behind the bed as they are close to your head.

● **Invest in EMF protection** Giawellness.com has a unique shielding technology that is patented in the USA. Their products for cell phones, PCs, TV sets and routers have been tested by a variety of laboratories and universities. The Hippocrates Health Institute has developed the H360, which claims to be the only EMF device to fully protect you in a 360 degree radius. www.hippocrateshealthinstitute.com

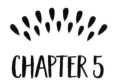

CHAPTER 5

THE SKULL IS NOT A SEALED BOX

*'A human mind was built for contact with similar minds.
It should, in fact, it must, think about what is going on
around it; for if it is shut up in a thick, dark, bony box of a
skull, it will always stay in that condition known as 'status
quo'; and grow up antagonistic to all surroundings.'*

ERNEST VINCENT WRIGHT, AUTHOR

As we have seen in Chapter 1, your brain is not a self-contained unit, safely protected, tucked away inside your head. The skull protects it but it's not a sealed box, instead there are access points directly into it from the world outside. The spinal cord may be protected by the vertebrae, but it reaches up into your brain. Your eyes are a pair of windows into your brain, and your nose, mouth and ears also offer the opportunity for outside interference. Each of these entry points has the potential to affect your brain – for better or worse.

Neuroscience now shows a clear link between the function of the ears, eyes and motor senses on your brain. They work closely together, integrating messages to and from the brain, which in turn coordinates and directs your body according to the clarity of the messages received and its ability to react to them. Develop a problem in any of these routes in and those messages will be compromised, and the brain will be correspondingly affected. The brain and sight, speech, sound and movement are so interconnected that when one sensory pathway stops working optimally, the function of the brain as a whole goes down with it. So, brain-related diseases can not only affect your vision, hearing and movement, for example, but conversely, difficulties with sight, sound, posture, balance, coordination or movement can adversely affect your brain, leading to concentration and attention problems and poor visual memory.

Inside your mouth

'The entire jawbone (upper and lower jaw) has become for most of us a toxic waste dump'

Max Daunderer MD

The metals used by dentists can make your brain sick. The area inside your mouth, your palate, is made of tissue and muscle, and can be penetrated more easily than the bone-hard, outer protective sheath that is your skull. Underneath your palate sit your 32 teeth. Their outer casing may be the hardest substance in your body, but they are encased in gums, which are the home of a multitude of minuscule bugs that live and thrive in the fluid in your mouth, the saliva.

Your toxic teeth

Anyone with a less than perfectly functioning brain needs to consider the potential danger lurking in their teeth. If I had to choose one single topic in the book to bring to your attention, this would be it. Have you ever considered what's gone into your mouth over the years? Fillings, bridges, implants, root canals or crowns? Dentists use a wide variety of metals in the work – you may have a combination of thallium, gold, titanium, mercury, palladium, nickel, aluminium, tin, or more in your teeth and jawbone. Most of these are a danger to the human body, and in combination can be lethal to your brain. Toxic metals are one of the few things that the body cannot get rid of on its own. Most of us have had repeated dental work done from a young age and rising levels of toxicity can show itself in physical symptoms, many of which are related to the brain.

The metals in your mouth can change the pH of your saliva, and, just like a car battery, in an aqueous solution can create a damagingly acidic environment and chemical corrosion that can cause problems. Implants rust and break down. A study of 132 patients found that eye problems, hearing, headaches, depression, feeling tearful, sensitivity to smells, metal taste in mouth, jaw pains, dry mouth, salivation and gum pains, sinusitis, tongue tremor and bad breath all improve considerably when amalgam is removed.[1] Small metal particles from the dental work travel throughout the body, lodging in your organs and bones,[2] and can penetrate your brain. Electromagnetic currents can disturb your meridians and energy flow, triggering allergic and immune reactions. Are you unable to find the cause of your brain issues – be it Alzheimer's or Parkinson's disease, for example? Have you ever thought that it could be metal that fills your cells at every level with toxicity.[3] Get rid of those metals though, and general health and brain benefits often result.

What is in a filling?

In 2008, the US Food and Drug Administration (FDA) said: 'Some individuals have an allergy or sensitivity to mercury or the other components of dental amalgam (such as silver, copper, or tin)... [which] might cause these individuals to develop oral lesions or other contact reactions.' But how would you know in advance if you had an allergy? Dentists rarely test their patients before working in their mouths. In addition, until fairly recently, fillings contained large amounts of mercury. We know now that it can be a trigger for both physical and mental health problems. A Taiwanese study found that women with amalgam fillings (containing mercury alongside other metals) were more than twice as likely to develop Alzheimer's disease.[4] The World Health Organisation considers it to be one of the 10 most dangerous chemicals for human health and states on its website that even the smallest amount of mercury exposure can cause serious issues, affecting almost all our body systems – immunity, digestion, nervous system, kidneys, eyes, skin and lungs. Recent research has shown that MRI scanners significantly increase the release of mercury. And yet many of us in the UK still have mercury fillings.

Your teeth sit directly under your brain and there is no dense bone barrier to protect it from any toxins coming from that direction. Mercury not only triggers inflammation, but it also deteriorates as it ages. Continual grinding breaks through the seal that originally held the mercury in check and allows a fine mist of particles to be released. This invades the softer palate, eventually penetrating the tissues of your brain. With mercury poisoning, your brain struggles to function. Memory problems and impaired cognition are just some of the symptoms, alongside headaches and mood changes such as increased irritability, depression and anxiety.[5]

Root canals, implants and crowns

Mercury fillings are just the tip of the iceberg. Many of us have had a tooth in trouble, where the decision had to be made to save it or replace it. Have you ever had root-canal treatment, or was a tooth capped with a crown? Like fillings, crowns and root canal treatments can themselves sometimes be a root cause of ill health. Do you know what your crown(s) is/are made of, or what sort of cement holds them in place?

And there can be problems with root extraction too. If your dentist doesn't clean out and disinfect the canal completely when they remove it, infection can set in under the treated tooth, which often doesn't show up even with an X-ray. Toxins then flood your system, causing unexpected problems and sometimes, eventually, serious disease. Implants can further weaken an already stressed organ.

What is your implant made of?

If you went for an implant, consider what it is made of. A whopping 95 per cent of them are made of titanium alloys. Are you allergic to titanium? You can find out with a home test. Official statistics say that only 0.6 per cent of us are allergic to it, but if you're one of the unlucky few, might your health issues be related? Titanium corrodes over time[6] – effectively, it can rust – which causes all sorts of problems. Miniscule amounts of metal flake off, and pus can build up – your body's reaction to an invading substance – causing inflammation. Tired all the time? It may be your body using most of its energy to keep a lid on your toxic teeth, not leaving much over to manage the rest of you. Not the onset of dementia after all, but the result of toxic dentistry. Remove the metals and the research shows that inflammation reduces and goes away.

Did you know...? The titanium conundrum

Titanium is widely used in medicine and is considered to be a safe material. Numerous studies support this, but recently more evidence is emerging that points to the possibility that it has side effects and can be a trigger for cognitive damage. Allergic reaction and corrosion of the metal are now well documented. Although the links to chronic disease are less well studied, surgeons and dentists report infections, neuropathy, pain, and bone reabsorption connected to it. Radiotherapy and titanium implants do not react well together either. This is a controversial topic, but still one it's worth looking into if radiotherapy has been offered to you.

Periodontal disease

Infections in the jaw can cause a bacterial overload in your mouth. The bacteria then enter your bloodstream through the gums, and the escapees attach themselves to fatty plaques in the bloodstream, causing a build-up on your blood vessel walls. This creates blockages and triggers an inflammatory response that causes swelling, reduces blood flow and increases the risk of blood clots. The bacteria can travel onwards to affect all parts of the body, including the brain. Chronic periodontitis has been shown to cause similar damage in the brain, clogging the brain's blood vessels and impairing memory.

Did you know... About metal braces?

Often fixed in your mouth for several years, braces are usually made of stainless steel, and an alloy of nickel, copper and titanium. Nickel is a known carcinogen, but is still used in modern day dentistry, up close to your brain. It commonly triggers allergic reactions in human tissue.

Action plan

Your brain problems may be linked to the condition of your teeth and gums. Put dental research high on your list and you may very well get your health back in hand.

- **Establish your metal load** Take a urine elements test to assess your loading. You can buy kits on the internet, for example, from www.biolab.co.uk. They can assess your urine and give you a list of your metal readings for, amongst others, lead, mercury, cadmium, arsenic, copper, aluminium and nickel. If your levels are high, and you don't take action, they will continue to build in your body, exacerbating existing health issues, and possibly causing new ones as time goes by.

- **Find out if you are allergic to any metals** Establish which metals, if any, your body reacts to. There are two tests you can do.

  The Melisa test (www.melisa.org) is the world's most in-depth metal allergy blood test. It looks at your immune response and will tell you exactly which metals you are allergic to, so if you have serious health issues and suspect metals in your body this is the one to choose. It was invented by Professor Vera Stajkal, in conjunction with the Karolinska Institute, Sweden, whose work has established the link between metal hypersensitivity and the development of chronic disease and autoimmune issues. [7]

  The Acumen test looks at cell signalling response and tests for heavy metals, plastics, pesticides, skincare products, medications and other toxins. Developed by Dr John McLaren-Howard, the acumen test identifies which toxins may be stuck to your DNA, switching off any genes in the process. Contact Acumen medical 01398 332437, or Acumenlabs.net

- **Detoxify yourself** This may take months, or even years, as metals are one of the substances the body cannot release by itself. Zeolite, a mineral substance made from volcanic ash, helps remove chemicals and pollutants. Supplements come in liquid form and work by binding toxins such as mercury, lead, cadmium and arsenic, absorbing them, then excreting them out of your body, detoxifying all your body's cells, including the brain cells. Take supplements for several months. Test your urine, above, before you start and again afterwards. Liquidzeolitecompany.com

- **Book a far-infrared (FIR) sauna** This is another effective way of detoxing metals.

- **Make an appointment to see a biological dentist** Ask them about the safe removal and replacement of dental amalgam. You can book in for a check-up, then make up your mind later, once you have done your research. The British Society for Mercury-free Dentistry has lists of approved practitioners. Many are members of the International Academy of Oral Medicine and Toxicology.

- **Bin your fluoride toothpaste** In high concentrations, fluoride can damage the brain, kidneys and thyroid, and there is no research that shows it is effective in protecting against cavities.

- **Drink a 'green' smoothie every morning** Make a celery and cucumber smoothie, adding a small bunch each of coriander (cilantro) and parsley, and two tablespoons of sage. This is a safe and gentle, yet effective, metal detox.

● **Drink silica-rich Acilis water** Drinking 1 litre (34 floz) a day for three months has been shown in tests to reduce levels of DNA-damaging aluminium and other metals (silicawaters.com). Research by Professor Chris Exley, Keele University, UK, has shown that the silica in the form of soluble silicic acid in this water enters the bloodstream and captures aluminium deposits, removing them through the urine. In doing so it re-energises the liver, kidneys and auto-immune system. For further information read the article on reboothealth.co.uk/Acilis water.

Your ears

If the eyes are the windows to your soul, the ears are the gateway to your brain. Research at the Department of Speech Language and Hearing Science at the University of Colorado, USA, suggests that there may be a direct correlation between hearing loss, brain decline and the development of dementia. They carried out a study in which they attached sensors to the heads of participants to measure the way their brains responded to different degrees of hearing loss when compared to people with normal hearing. What they found was that when hearing loss happened, the brain rewired itself, handing the areas that usually deal with hearing over to sections that process touch or vision. However, they also found that this transfer had a negative effect on cognition, so that even with a mild hearing loss, the hearing parts of the brain became weaker.[8]

One in three people over the age of 60 develop some degree of hearing loss. Yet statistics show that fewer than a quarter of the people who need hearing aids actually have them. On average, people wait seven years to get help, which is a long time for your brain to be in decline. So, don't put off having hearing aids for too long – your hearing and your brain will remain stronger for longer. A French study examining cochlear implants in the elderly revealed that cognitive skills, thinking and memory improved as speech comprehension improved.[9] In other words, a neuroplastic adjustment took place within their brains to reverse any damage that had been done as a result of their hearing loss.

The healing power of sound

The power of sound is vastly underestimated. Sound travels into your brain via your ears and can be used to heal – or it can harm – both your brain and the cells of your body. Sound can be powerful, so be aware of its effects and use it carefully. It is made up of combinations of different frequencies, and is measured in hertz (or Hz). The higher the sound, or pitch, the faster the vibration; the lower the sound, the slower the vibration.

Sound travels through the air in waves and can influence other vibrations it comes into contact with, and rebalance cells. 'Om', the sacred primordial chant sound, vibrates at the frequency of 432Hz, and calms both the nervous system and the mind. The 12th-century monks at Cluny Abbey, France, famously used music and chanting to successfully heal their patients. Now, of course, we know there is a scientific explanation: sound waves influence brain waves.

The type of sound healing that will be most restorative for you depends on your brain state. Those who have difficulty focusing have been found to benefit from beta- and gamma-targeting sound, while anyone who has trouble relaxing will find it easier to switch off with theta, alpha or delta waves. You can download specific brainwave sound meditations online, and try out one of the many binaural beats, pulsating rhythms that your brain 'makes' itself as it synthesises other sounds.

Music and sound have different effects on different people and can affect your mental state and body function. What soothes one person may trigger difficult memories for another. Think about the noise you live with every day, and reflect on what it could be doing to your brain (and the other organs of your body) as the cells and tissues absorb the energies of sound on a daily basis. Sound can alter your blood pressure, pulse, breathing rhythm, and release pain and stress. Low-frequency sounds can stress your body without you even being aware they are there. Most of us spend considerable amounts of time listening to music without any idea of its potential impact. Loud piercing noises – the whistle of a train, the rumble of the underground train, the roar of traffic or the sound of a jet surging down the runway – put stress both on both the body and the mind. Make sure the sounds you choose to listen to inspire and soothe rather than stress you.

Action plan

- **Book a hearing test** If there is any hearing loss buy hearing aids.

- **Clean out your ears** Talk to your doctor as they can do this for you. Never try to clean wax from your ears with a cotton bud as you can damage the eardrum inside.

- **Do your own personalised 'sound check'** Go through your usual music playlist and weed out the sounds that don't uplift you mentally. Make a power playlist for the times when you need energy or happy distraction from pain or difficult feelings, and a quieter playlist for when you want to calm your emotions.

- **Book in for some acupuncture** There are specific points that relate to the ears, which can boost your hearing.

Music can alter your brain waves

Music triggers the release of endorphins, improving mood and lessening pain. The slower the wave the calmer the feeling it engenders. Baroque music and New Age music shift consciousness from beta to alpha waves, while shamanic drumming, singing bowls and the didgeridoo can move you into theta states – the type your brain enters during deep meditation and sleep. Many alternative practitioners believe that musical tones relate to specific meridians and organs of the human body and can be used to strengthen and heal them.

To help concentration try some Mozart, which is proven to improve focus.

For serenity, listen to calm, peaceful music, for example, Gregorian chants. This will slow your thoughts, calm your emotions, and help clear your brain of distraction.

Be mindful of 'stressful' music Blood pressure levels can rise 10 per cent under the influence of loud noise as it releases stress hormones. Loud rock music, for example, can jar all the body systems and bring on headaches.

Sound can ease muscle pain This is really true. Lower frequencies of 40–66Hz relax the lower half of your body, whilst higher frequencies relax the top half of the body and your brain.

Your spine and brainstem connection

The very first parts of your body to form are your spinal cord and your brain stem – they are the master controllers that regulate all the functioning of your body. Next comes every other section of the body, along with the middle (emotion and memory) and frontal (higher cognitive functions) parts of the brain (see page 19). Together, the brain and spinal cord form your central nervous system (CNS), and everything is connected to this central core. The CNS is connected to the nerves of the peripheral nervous system, via circuits that stretch the length and breadth of your body and control every function automatically.

The peripheral nervous system has two parts: the sympathetic and parasympathetic systems. The sympathetic nervous system speeds things up and stimulates the body's fight-flight response. If you are, for example, over-stressed, you are likely to have an overactive sympathetic nervous system. The parasympathetic nervous system, in contrast, slows everything down and rebalances the aroused sympathetic part. The latter is responsible for controlling the body at rest and activities such as meditation, sex, breathwork or listening to relaxing music will help stimulate it.

It is perhaps not surprising then that how well your brain works is due in no small part to the correct alignment of your spine. Research indicates that adjustments by osteopaths and chiropractors can improve brain function, and especially the functioning of your prefrontal cortex, which controls decision making, focus and intelligence. So, if you are suffering from brain fog, anxiety, depression or frequent headaches, your back may be a good place to start. Chiropractic and osteopathy, in short, improve the connections between your brain and your body.[10]

A study carried out by Patricia Brennan PhD, in 1991, found that immune response was improved following chiropractic treatment – the numbers of natural killer (NK) cells, which destroy damaged and cancerous cells, increased.[11] Research by Ronald Pero, chief of cancer prevention research at New York's Preventive Medicine Institute, observed the immune strength of those who had had chiropractic treatment over a five-year period was 200 per cent greater than the control group who had no treatments. It was also 400 per cent stronger than those with cancer or other serious diseases.

The atlas bone is like a 'fuse box'

The spinal column that surrounds and protects the spinal cord is made up of a series of 33 bones, or vertebrae. The ultimate secret to brain health may lie in one simple adjustment to what could be the most important bone in the body, the first vertebra, which sits directly under your skull and at the top of the brain stem, known as C (cervical) 1, or the atlas bone. Each time you have an accident, whether it was falling off a bike at the age of five, or off a horse or ladder later on, or even if you simply trip over, there is a risk of the atlas going out of alignment. Whiplash, following a car accident, for example, virtually guarantees it, as can a particularly difficult birth. When the doctor puts hands or forceps around a baby's head during delivery and pulls, and perhaps twists as well, the atlas can be dislodged, which creates problems from that point onwards.

If the atlas bone becomes misaligned, your brain stem can be constricted, which prevents your CNS from functioning optimally. Research shows that even pressure as light as the weight of a small coin on the spinal cord can diminish nerve flow up to 60 per cent. This interference can mean healing messages simply stop flowing to all parts of your body, and particularly to your brain. Cerebrospinal fluid doesn't flow up to the brain fully, the discs between the vertebrae begin to degenerate, blood flow is restricted, and the nerves begin to malfunction, affecting both your immune system and your brain, creating a cascade effect throughout the body preventing normal signals running as they should. The power of both body, and mind diminishes. Realigning your atlas is a safe, gentle procedure with no cracking or popping of the spine. Research has shown that HIV and immunity markers can go down after an atlas correction,[12] while scoliosis is improved and high blood pressure reduced by 30 per cent.[13]

Action plan

- **Consider chiropractic or osteopathic treatment** It may take a few sessions. Upper cervical chiropractic is a unique technique that involves aligning the atlas bone. Once any disturbance is sorted, your brain's messages begin to flow again and both body and mind can heal.

- **Take up Alexander technique, Pilates or yoga** These can all help strengthen your back and improve your posture and they can all be done on your own at home, with the help of a YouTube tutorial.

- **Book a course of Rolfing** This is a therapy that rebalances the body by lengthening the fascia (soft tissues surrounding organs) and improving and correcting the muscles and structure of the body, freeing the spine. In the process, blockages that may affect the optimal functioning of the brain are released. Named after its inventor Ida Rolf, and much loved by ballet dancers, it involves deep manual therapy over a series of ten sessions.

● **Book in for acupuncture** I had an epidural during my first daughter's birth, and went repeatedly afterwards to the doctors complaining of a fuzzy brain, to no avail. One session of acupuncture and my brain came storming back – I could literally feel it unblocking as I lay on the table. Try it for yourself.

● **Reset your temporomandibular joint (TMJ)** You have a joint on either side of your head that attaches your jawbone to your skull. Misalignment, for example, by a blow to the head, falling over, whiplash or dentistry work where your mouth is forced open for a long period of time, can have an effect on your brain. It can distort the signals it sends and receives, or not send them at all. Headaches, clicking in your jaw and tightness in your neck and shoulders may all be indicators. Dr Shabir Pandor offers courses on how to reset it from his clinic in London's Harley Street (0207 580 1076).

The eyes: your mind's eye...

'Seeing is largely a function of the mind, and only partly a function of the eyes. There are 80 to 110 million rods and 4 to 5 million cones with which the retina senses light. A billion images are produced in the retina every minute. But the brain can't assimilate all these images: it's selective, and determines how much of a picture you will or won't see. It also determines how clear or how fuzzy your vision will be.'

MEIR SCHNEIDER, HOLISTIC HEALER

Vision is a brain process, though we rarely consider the connection between our eyes and our brain. It is an automatic, or non-conscious, process, which happens every second of every day. Around one third of your brain is devoted to processing what you see – distinguishing between distance and depth, recognising faces, objects and colours. All of this is carried out without any help from your conscious mind; your conscious mind then tells you what your brain has already worked out. Vision and sight are part and parcel of the same whole – sight is the ability to see, whereas vision deals with brain function (mainly concentration and attention) and motor skills. When your eyes weaken, so too do your brain and your body.

Our eyes feed information directly to the brain, which acts instantaneously on that information. When you arrive in a new place, meet a new person, or decide to do a certain thing, your eyes are working overtime, continually assessing, judging and feeling. Your actions, coordinated by your brain, are the direct results of those initial perceptions. So, what happens if your eyes are not in top condition? The messages your brain receives will not be as exact either, and your brain's responses will be slower than they should be.

From the moment you are born, everything you experience – your thoughts, beliefs and feelings – are based on what you have seen and how you have chosen to interpret it. There is more than a metre of nerve fibres leaving each eye – around 70 per cent of the sensory nerves in the body – passing on and filtering innumerable pieces of information, which are then acted on by the brain. Many of the eye's nerve fibres are linked to the middle part of the cortex, to the centres that manage balance, coordination and movement, touch and spatial perception. The quality of your sight, therefore, affects the way your brain works, the way you think, remember and perceive the world around you. Your vision organises the way you stand and move, as well as balance and how you relate to the space that surrounds you.

What you feed your eyes on – figuratively and literally – has been linked to brain function and health. Like your gut, your eyes have their own microbiome, a specific collection of fungi, bacteria and viruses that live on your eyeballs. And, like your gut, it can go out of balance, triggering eye infections and diseases and affecting the function of your brain. Think carefully before taking antibiotics for an eye infection. Not only do they not affect viruses, but they may be destroying your good eye microbes as well.[14]

Science has identified a clear connection between the health of the eyes and the health of your brain. If there's something wrong with your eyes and vision, there is likely to be a malfunction in your brain. Think of the lens of a camera. When you try to get it to focus on something that is too close for its usual range, the autofocus will struggle, repeatedly zooming in and out. When your vision flags, your eyes are continually doing something similar, all day long, exhausting the brain and your body in the process. Parkinson's and Lyme diseases, multiple sclerosis and brain injury are all conditions that affect visual processing, and the harder you try to focus the more your symptoms increase.

If you become aware of vision problems, pay attention, because your brain will also be affected. Around 68 per cent of people in the UK suffer from some sort of impaired vision, and in the USA that figure is 75 per cent. Before the arrival of the tsunami of technology that overwhelms us today, we used our eyes more extensively. Nowadays, our range of vision is more or less set, at a fixed distance from a tablet, phone or computer. And the more time you spend glued to your screens, the less your eye muscles can flex and stay strong. In addition, the 'blue' light that emanates from LEDs, fluorescent lights, and the endless screens and devices, is detrimental to eye health. It causes a build-up of free radicals on the retinas, and damages the rods and cones behind them.

Action plan

- **Book an eye test** An optometrist will not only check your vision to find out whether you need glasses, or make sure that your current prescription is correct, but also undertake a thorough eye health check. Visual field assessment (VFA) is used to detect the onset of eye disease, which may correlate with a weakening of parts of the brain that control motor and sensory perception. Loss of peripheral vision can lead to difficulty with mobility and orientation, and with reaching and grasping, and lead to an increased risk of falling.[15]

- **Take a visual contrast sensitivity (VCS) test** This can be done online for a small charge at www.vcstest.com. You will be shown a series of images of decreasing contrast and be asked to record contrast levels where you can – or cannot – identify specific patterns, shapes, or objects. A poor result may indicate neurological weakening. Contact with mould (see pages 75–77) can damage nerve cells, causing a reduction in contrast vision. However, this can be managed and reversed if the mould toxins are removed.

- **Take an eye-specific supplement** Choose one that contains lutein, zeaxanthin and meso-zeaxanthin.[16] Tests show they can improve eyesight as well as protect the macula from slow, age-related macular degeneration.

- **Put blue light protecting screens on your devices** Adding a protective screen to the surfaces of your mobile phone, tablet or computer protects your eyes from damage.

- **Include omega-3 fatty acids in your diet** A deficiency is associated with poor night vision and problems with visual, spatial and attention processing. (See also Chapter 7.)

- **Treat dry eye** Take omega-6 in the form of clary sage oil – put one drop in each eye and take it orally too.

- **Try light therapy** Low-level light therapy (LLLT) significantly improves vision in 95 per cent of eyes with cataracts and 97 per cent of those without cataracts.[17] Brain photobiomodulation, where a device is directed at your head or clipped on to the inside of your nose and to beam near infrared light towards the brain, has been found to improve cognitive ability[18] (see also Chapter 11). A 2018 review of photobiomodulation found that it had: *'the potential to treat a wide range of brain disorders including Parkinson's, depression, anxiety, autism and PTSD'.*[19]

- **Book in for alternative treatments** Low-level electrical microcurrents applied to the eyelids can help both 'wet' and 'dry' macular degeneration. Low-level laser therapy can be used to treat diabetic retinopathy, amblyopia (or lazy eye) and age-related macular degeneration. Acupuncture can improve blurry or distorted vision and dry eyes, and repair damaged visual pathways, and is effective for symptoms of macular degeneration, optic neuropathy and some types of glaucoma.

- **Look at cannabis options** Ask your doctor about these treatments – certain cannabinoids have been found to be effective in treating glaucoma – THCa in particular (see reference section, page 271).

> ### Did you know... About the OcuShield?
>
> This is an inexpensive film screen developed by an optician concerned about the connection between blue light and the onset of age-related macular degeneration. It fits precisely, and invisibly, over your smart phone or tablet screen, cutting out all damaging UV rays. Used correctly you can read on your tablet late at night without the blue light affecting your ability to sleep.

Your nose knows

The sense of smell is closely linked to the processes of both thinking and breathing. There are many studies on the benefits of breath-based meditation on the brain. Where once this was thought of as new-age junk science, there is now a widely accepted scientific consensus that conscious breathing is deeply connected to brain function.

Studies on rats have shown that when they sniff, the air they breathe in stimulates their brain activity, triggering neurons in the olfactory bulb to communicate with the hippocampus, the part of the brain that stores memories. A recent research project at the Karolinska Institute, Sweden, looked to see if there was a similar brain connection in humans, triggered by breathing in through our mouths.[20] Two dozen healthy young male and female volunteers inhaled 12 different scents from small vials held to their noses. The subjects were asked to memorise each scent – some of the smells were familiar, like the essence of orange, while others were obscure. They went through this process on two occasions. For one, they sat quietly for an hour immediately after the sniffing, with their noses clipped shut to prevent nasal breathing; on the other, they sat for an hour with tape over their mouths to prevent oral breathing. According to the researchers' hypothesis, during each hour their brains should have been consolidating memories of the smells in the hippocampus. After each hour, the volunteers were exposed to some of the same scents and some new ones, then asked to determine whether an odour had been sniffed earlier. The participants were found to be consistently better at recognising smells if they breathed through their noses during the quiet hour. Mouth breathing resulted in fuzzier recall and more incorrect answers. The conclusion was that nasal breathing enhanced memory consolidation, whereas mouth breathing alone did not have the same effect; it by-passed the olfactory bulb, so did not trigger the same neuronal cascade.

Brain-boosting aromatherapy

Aromatherapy is a great way of stimulating healing through the sense of smell. Used correctly it can be a powerful adjunct for rebooting your brain. Scents in essential oils stimulate parts of the brain that control memories and emotion and can affect other physical issues too. Northumbria University, UK, carried out a study with a group of elderly participants and found that merely being in a room diffused with the smell of rosemary boosted memory scores by 15 per cent.[21] Lavender oil, meanwhile, has been found not only to reduce symptoms of depression, anxiety and insomnia, but also to increase production of relaxing theta and alpha brain waves.[22]

Action plan

- ➤ **Book in for yoga sessions** Learning yoga pranayama breathing techniques will oxygenate your brain and clear your nasal passages.

- ➤ **Try light** The Vielight 810 is a small device that you clip onto the side of your nose to beam NIR light up your nasal passages, boosting your mental function (see also Chapter 11).

● **Try brain-boosting essential oils** All of the following oils have been found in studies to improve different aspects of brain function. Place a few drops of your chosen oil on a tissue and inhale it at regular intervals.

Lavender reduces stress, worry, disruptive behaviour and uplifts mood.

Clary sage reduces stress and worry, improves memory and learning.

Sandalwood improves mental focus and attention span, reduces worry and calms disruptive behaviour.

Rosemary improves memory and focus.

Frankincense lowers levels of stress and worry and stimulates memory and learning.

Lemon balm calms agitation and improves communication and brain function as well as decreasing difficult behaviour.

Peppermint increases oxygen levels in the brain and boosts energy. It is also anti-inflammatory.

Ylang ylang, patchouli, marjoram and vetiver have been found to reduce agitation and disturbed behaviour in dementia patients.

Jasmine has been found to balance the central nervous system, increasing beta waves in the brain and triggering feelings of wellbeing.[23]

The tip of your tongue

Your tongue is closely linked to your brain, with the nerves on the very tip directly connecting to the brain stem. The brain stem controls the muscles and the body, directing balance and integrating motor and sensory information so that it flows smoothly, passing messages directly from the brain to the body. Tongue stimulation, influencing the brain via the tongue nerve pathways, looks like becoming an influential treatment for neurological issues.

Action plan

- **Research treatment with a pulsed electromagnetic field (PEMF) machine** A recent study has found that stimulating the tongue with a PEMF machine activates the neural network in the brain in charge of balance and can help multiple sclerosis patients improve their muscle control. The same technique was applied to patients who had had a stroke, and those with Parkinson's and loss of sight, with similar success.[24] (See also Chapter 11.)

- **Book an acupuncture session** The tongue is where two of the most important meridians in the body meet. Acupuncture can normalise the energy centres situated in the tongue, and brain fog and brain-related memory issues can be treated by boosting energy flow in the area.

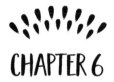

CHAPTER 6

EMOTIONS AND THEIR EFFECT ON THE BRAIN

'The mind is like a house... thoughts which the owner no longer wishes to display, or those which arouse painful memories, are thrust out of sight, and consigned to attic or cellar...'

MARGARET ATWOOD, AUTHOR

Our past is always and inevitably part of our present. It has formed who we are and how we got to where we are today. We've all had experiences that have been psychologically highly significant. Childhood traumas, disappointments and upsets may be very difficult to process, and the brain does not forget about them whatever we do in an attempt to move on – instead it stores them as a reminder of where danger lies. Present-day stressors can often re-activate deep-set patterns and beliefs linked to those formative experiences and memories.

Problems arise when present-day stress creates psychological responses that impede your ability to think clearly. They stir up the emotional baggage and bring it into the 'now' in ways that sometimes makes it very difficult to sort out, irrespective of whether the particular emotions are appropriate to the current situation. When this happens, you may find that you can't think efficiently, clearly or integratively, because your brain is overrun with anxious or depressive thoughts. But because anxiety and depression are so prevalent (one in four people in the UK will experience a mental health disorder in any given year[1]), many of us come to accept them, and the associated impairment of our brain function, as a fact of life.

Accepting chronic stress as a normal way of life is not healthy. Low mood and listlessness can manifest as brain fog and lack of mental energy and it's easy to become preoccupied by the surface symptoms rather than their deeper causes. Similarly, anxiety can take over, forcing you to think in unhelpful loops or up blind alleys, leading you to doubt not only your own mind but your capacity for high-level, analytical thought. Before you can tackle the root causes of these brain, and life-hampering conditions, it is helpful to understand something of the recesses of the non-conscious mind.

Consciousness and the two minds that rule us

The mind is like an iceberg. The part we are all aware of is our 'conscious' mind, the tip of the iceberg – the bit that is visible above the water. This is the part of you that you are aware of day-to-day. It includes your consciously held ideas and beliefs, the part of you that is endlessly chatting and commenting. It decides if something is right or wrong, it judges and discriminates, it plans for the future, and examines the past. But it bases all of its decisions on the non-conscious 'information' upon which everything in its experience is predicated (see opposite): the visible tip of the iceberg could not be there if it was not being supported by everything underneath it. The conscious mind acts rather like the announcer on a stage, publicly putting forth the story that your brain has already, long before, decided to tell. It is the voice of your intuition and of your deepest beliefs.

Your non-conscious mind is the vast and unseen hidden part of the iceberg. It holds about 90 per cent of your brain's power and is always on duty, 24/7, efficiently managing whatever behaviour is required at a specific moment, without the need of conscious supervision. For example, this is the part of your brain that manages to drive a car without thinking; it takes over from the conscious brain once it has learned the initial skill. This is also the part that learns from and stores past experiences. It has the potential for changing or re-interpreting the past because of added circumstance, but sometimes fails to do so without conscious instruction and intention.

The danger here is that in setting up strategies to keep you 'safe', the brain's primary task is to make the best adaptations it can from its own particular storehouse of experience. It doesn't necessarily take into consideration the more recent facts when circumstances have changed over time – that you grew up and learned to stand up for yourself, that the threat changed, that a difficult person died or moved out of your life. Unless you regularly upgrade the programmes that have been running you since childhood, they will remain in place even though they may no longer be nearly so relevant to your life now.

Subliminal thoughts and beliefs created from your past experiences run like a recording inside you – 24 hours a day. If, non-consciously, you have decided that you can't do something, then that 'I can't do it' recording plays night and day, and not even a 60-minute 'conscious' daily visualisation, affirmation, or positive thinking session will be able to make even a dent in the 23 hours of subliminal negative thinking.

To free yourself from persistent negative thoughts, you need to tackle them head on. The exercises in this chapter will help you do just that. But be aware, however, that if 'you', the fundamental, absolutely central control mechanism set up by your deepest self, *really really* doesn't want to change, no amount of coercive, or otherwise, practice will make it happen.

The iceberg of the mind

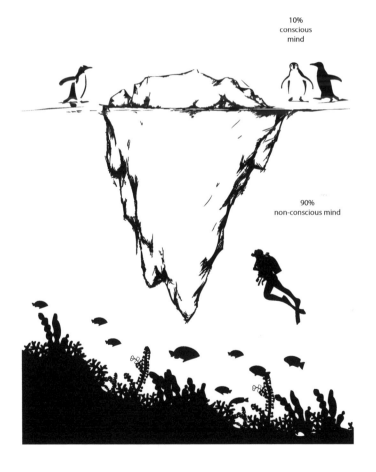

Did you know...?

The non-conscious mind is incredible, it:

- has 50,000–70,000 thoughts a day

- processes 20,000 environmental stimuli per second

- is in charge of 100,000 chemical reactions per cell per second in the body

- processes 20 million pieces of information per second[2]

The power of positive thought

Thinking positively can be very hard when you are feeling overwhelmed and stressed. But there are very good reasons why it's important to try. As the developmental biologist Bruce Lipton explains in his remarkable book, *The Biology of Belief*, specific strong feelings like grief, anger, revenge, fear or depression trigger strong associated chemicals, such as cortisol and adrenaline, which, if released into your bloodstream daily over a long period of time, can have a detrimental impact on your brain.

But changing your way of thinking can help you to take back control of your mental health and your brain function and you will feel good. Choosing to behave and think in ways that flood your body with positive feelings (gratitude, joy, peace and love) on a daily basis has a powerful physiological impact on the wellbeing of your body (and brain) because of the chemicals associated with those feelings. But before we explore some of the ways to tackle and disrupt underlying negative beliefs and retrain yourself to think more productively and with greater focus, let's look at the way that the two most common mental health conditions – anxiety and depression – impact on our emotional and cognitive function.

Anxiety can take over

When your fight-flight response is habituated, or when worry and rumination take over, as can happen when you are overwhelmed with fear or anxiety, it can become much harder to engage in big-picture thinking and imagination. The brain is either doing its best to prioritise its primary fear response at the expense of other processes, or it is so caught up in unproductive overthinking, that clarity and focus become impossible. In short, anxiety is characterised by intrusive thoughts and bodily sensations that take up precious mental resources, and divert energy and attention needed elsewhere. But, being the adaptive organ that it is, the brain is doing its best based on your experience to-date (which is all it has got to go on). So how could you help it do better?

Neuroimaging studies have shown that in anxiety disorders where panic and panic attacks are present they are characteristic of an overactive 'limbic' brain, particularly of the amygdala.[3] Interestingly though, more generalised anxiety disorders, characterised by worrying and rumination, have been found to correlate to hyperactivity in the pre-frontal cortex itself,[4] indicating that when it comes to anxiety, there are a range of presentations, causes and characteristics, which makes generalisation hard.

However, we do know that generalised anxiety disorder is associated with a decline in working memory function and selective attention ability.[5] This is not surprising as the energy available to the brain is being stretched to capacity, so it is not available for other purposes, however much more useful they might be. We also know that when anxious people receive treatment such as psychotherapy, exercise and meditation for anxiety, they show improvements in their brain function and mental wellbeing. This gives hope to anyone wanting to break free from the grip of anxiety – it really is possible to train yourself consciously to get your brain working differently, as you would like it to work, not just retrieve it from the depths of its non-conscious habits.

It is worth remembering, though, that whatever was happening when your anxiety responses were first established was likely to have been an appropriate adaptation at the time. The fact that the reaction has persisted is because your brain is doing its best to look after you. From your brain's point of view, it is better to stay in touch with what might mean danger, and to generalise that primary reaction, than to risk not seeing the danger. The problem is that when the brain does this it draws the energy supply from your higher mental functions, so they can't operate as they should.

Depression – impairs your ability to think straight

Depression is often triggered by a build-up of stress, or a one-off, overwhelming traumatic event (the death of a loved one or being made redundant, for example). It may feel impossible to move on from the initial sadness and hopelessness. The chemical changes in the brain with regard to three key neurotransmitters, dopamine, noradrenaline, and serotonin, are known to be characteristic of depression,[6] although their unique interrelation varies significantly from person to person.

When you are depressed it is harder to function. You can't think flexibly and laterally, and memory and reasoning are negatively affected. And, even if you seek medication, new evidence from a study of 1,000 depressed people by an international research team found that although drug treatments improved mood, they did little to nothing to improve the characteristic cognitive impairment of depression.[7] Depression is bad news for the long-term decline of the brain, too. A 2018 study found that depressed older adults were more than twice as likely to develop vascular dementia as their non-depressed peers, and 65 per cent more likely to develop Alzheimer's.[8]

The problem with the 'keep calm and carry on' approach

If you want to get to the bottom of the underlying emotional distress that may be causing anxiety or depression or may just be keeping you 'stuck', you need to face up to some uncomfortable feelings and memories that are perhaps very difficult to manage. Ask yourself: What aren't you dealing with? What bits of yourself are sabotaging your brain health, and emotional and intellectual function?

Your brain is always doing the best for you that it can; it just may lack the resources to be other than it is. When you can identify that you *want* to be different, that emotion carries that instruction directly to the 'Self', and the intention sets the way forward – the task of becoming different.

Stress: unload your brain's burden

Stress is the number one cause of mental exhaustion. It consumes energy voraciously and, unsurprisingly, it takes its toll on your brain function. Stress can drain more than 70 per cent of the blood from your frontal lobes – the area connected to thinking – depriving them of oxygen and impairing your ability to focus. A 2017 US study found that higher perceived stress correlated with higher levels of cognitive decline, most notably in episodic memory and visuospatial ability.[9] Another more recent study showed that when rats were stressed repeatedly, their memory was impaired.[10] Researchers identified specific 'mal-adaptions' to the stress in the brain that caused the decline in brain function.

Stress reactions start in the body, but manifest themselves in your mind as you try to make sense of what your body is trying to tell you. Everyday worries – about work or financial difficulties, traffic jams, personal relationships or even the everyday news on the radio and TV – trigger a build-up of stress. Through the mechanisms of perception – known as epigenetic influence – this in turn affects the physical brain, which is, of course, part of the body, but it has the special task of creating and managing 'mind'. Eventually, if the stress is not dealt with, you find yourself temporarily unable to think or function; it's rather like trying to drive in the fast lane of a motorway with the handbrake on.

Raised levels of cortisol, the hormone associated with stress, reduces the numbers of neurons in your hippocampus (the area that deals with learning, memory and emotional control) and destroys your mitochondria.[11] If you keep thinking the same negative thoughts, your cortisol will continue flowing, reducing your brain's cognitive function in the process. ***Changing your thoughts is therefore vital for brain health – do this and you can literally change your brain.***

Past and present stress counteract each other

We all deal with difficult experiences in different ways and what seems small and bearable to one person may feel like the end of the world to another. If, in the present, you can still remember, see and feel what happened many years earlier, then that event is still 'live' in your non-conscious mind, working to safeguard you. If that memory is proving unhelpful, it needs to be brought into your conscious mind, its value recognised, and then shifted into a different place in your system with different residual values attached to it. It's not a disorder or disease that you have, though you may feel very dis-ordered or dis-eased; it's simply that an earlier appropriate response is coming inappropriately into your present. Originally it was of value – just as, at the right time in your development, behaving as a child was exactly right. But now that the circumstances are different, adaptations are required. If the earlier experience signalled real danger, confusion or serious threat, your brain prefers to hang on to the experience – *just in case* – as your mind's priority is to protect you from perceived danger. Through our new understanding of brain plasticity and epigenetics, we now know, however, that you have the power to help your brain understand that there is no need to let it be part of the present any longer; it can let the old go.

Just how stressed are you?

Have a look at the inventory of life stresses chart below[12]. How many of these life events have happened to you in the last 12 months? Answering the questions and adding up your score will give you a fairly accurate picture of the stress you are under now.

Life event	Mean value
Death of a spouse/partner	100
Divorce	73
Separation from spouse/partner	65
Detention in jail or other institution	63
Death of a close family member	63
Major personal injury or illness	53
Marriage	50
Being fired from work	47
Reconciliation with spouse/partner	45
Retirement from work	45
Major change in the health or behaviour of family member	44

continued...

Pregnancy	40
Sexual difficulties	39
Gaining new family member (through birth, adoption, or older adult moving in)	39
Major business readjustment	39
Major change in financial position (either a lot better off or worse off)	38
Death of a close friend	37
Changing to a different line of work	36
Major change in number of arguments with spouse (either a lot more or a lot less than usual, regarding, for example, childrearing, personal habits etc.)	35
Taking on a mortgage or loan (for home or business)	31
Foreclosure on a mortgage or loan (for home or business)	30
Major change in responsibilities at work (either promotion or demotion)	29
Son or daughter leaving home (for example, for college, marriage, or employment)	29
Difficulties with your partner's family	29
Outstanding personal achievement	28
Spouse/partner beginning or stopping work outside the home	26
Beginning or ceasing formal schooling	26
Major change in living conditions (moving home, deterioration of neighbourhood or home)	25
Major revision to personal habits (e.g. quitting smoking/alcohol, changes to dress, manners or associations)	24
Troubles with your boss	23
Major changes to working hours or conditions	20
Changes in residence	20
Changing schools	20
Major change in usual type and/or amount of recreational activity	19

continued...

Major change in church activity (more or less than usual)	19
Major change in social activities (clubs, movies, visiting friends etc.)	18
Taking out a loan for a car, household furniture/appliances	17
Major change in sleeping habits (much more or much less than usual)	16
Major change in number of family get-togethers	15
Major change in eating habits (a lot more or less than usual, or very different mealtimes or surroundings)	15
Vacation	13
Major holiday	12
Minor violations (speeding or parking fines, disturbing the peace etc.)	11

Now add up your results

- **150 points or fewer** shows a relatively low amount of life change and a low susceptibility to stress-induced health breakdown.

- **150 to 300 points** indicates a 50 per cent chance of health breakdown in the next two years.

- **300 points or more** indicates an 80 per cent chance of health breakdown in the next two years.

While this is a good wake-up call, what about more deeply buried stresses and traumas in your past? In the rest of this chapter I will focus on a series of simple exploratory DIY tests, investigations and exercises to help you identify underlying unhelpful beliefs, dysfunctional thinking and habits that are standing in the way of you tapping into the restorative power of your brain.

Exercise 1: Create a de-stress route map

What would make your life more the one you want it to be, and minimise the stress you are under? The stresses of everyday life can seem to make you rush from pillar to post, and weeks, months and even years, pass in a flash. You may be 'surviving', but it can feel as if life is running you; you are not creating its content and direction.

Life rarely gives you the time to consciously consider what would give you the most satisfaction in the long term. Sit quietly and alone and take your time to consider what would really make your heart sing – might it be moving to a new home, travelling, finding a partner, changing job or getting a pet? Take as long as you need, let your mind pop the answers into your head. Write down your answers, in as much detail as possible. You may be surprised at what arises when you really listen to yourself.

The mind works on instructions, so once you are clear on where you want to go, and what changes are needed to make it happen, set this as a clear intention for your future, then repeat it to yourself constantly. This is a very different process from the misguided 'Mend my life' wish or 'My life will be fixed when...' This is a command that tells your mind that you already have what you wish for. Imagine the change in the present – for example the new buyers (of the flat you haven't been able to sell for months, because the message you are sending to your mind daily is 'the flat's not selling'), are asking which pieces of furniture they can buy.

The mind does exactly what it is told, always. It can't distinguish between reality and imagined reality. It merely follows the instructions it is given and does its best to deliver that instruction. Chaotic thoughts and negative messaging will deliver chaotic and negative results to your door. Similarly, a mental image of your new life, with your new brain imagined as clearly and specifically as you can, will deliver a concrete plan to you. Hold your future sense of yourself clearly before you, and before you know it, your life will move in a different direction.

Exercise 2: Write out your past stresses

To move past stresses out of your brain, try the next exercise. Get a notebook, then sit still (or even lie down) for a few minutes in a quiet room. Shut your eyes and ask your mind to send you images of anything that needs resolving; let memories and pictures flood your mind. They may all seem unconnected, but, of course, they are part of you, so are in fact very connected. People, places and things that you haven't thought of for years will come into your head, some of them seemingly insignificant, and some with unexpected clarity.

Write everything down – just use short headings that you can use to jog your memory later. It may be anything from when you fell off the sofa as a baby, Billy pushed you over in the playground when you were seven years old and everyone laughed at you, your first difficult day at secondary school, failing an exam, to ending your first relationship, losing your job, your dog dying, being left by a partner, or the death of a parent. The pressures of everyday life are endless and varied.

The list, and its length, will be different for everyone. Some people will focus on events from years ago, and others on more recent happenings. If you have been under a lot of stress recently, your recall for long-past events will be slower, but surprising connections will still appear. What is important is that you keep writing until no more pictures and memories come into your head; it doesn't matter how long that list becomes.

Each memory that is attached to escape/avoidance/survival emotions carries a portion of all the stress your system is experiencing and adds to your sense of psychological burden.

Bringing them into your conscious mind is the first step on the path to realising their past significance, and then releasing their current intrusive hold over you. Some will take more effort to re-organise than others. For the experiences and memories that affect you most deeply, long-term talking therapy may be required, but others can be worked through with simple self-directed exercises such as the ones in this chapter. A session or two of specific complementary therapies (as listed in Chapter 10) will also help you resolve problems that may have overburdened you for years.

Exercise 3: Home truths and life sentences

Our experiences of relationships can tell us a great deal about not just ourselves, but also our brains. Complete the following sentences on a piece of paper.

In my experience, most people are ....

I find women/men are ....
I have learned this because ....

And men/women, in my life, have ....
I have learned this because...

Families are ....
When I was a child, my family felt...

Friendships are..
because people ....

Look at your answers. Can you see themes developing in the way you experience other people, that you think people behave towards you, or in the 'truths' you hold about how people are? These experiences and thoughts can sometimes tell you more about yourself than about other people. Are you unwittingly seeking out friends and partners who confirm your unhelpful or unhealthy 'truths' about people? In what ways does this have a negative impact on you? Challenging and disrupting unhelpful beliefs is the first step on the way to taking more control over your relationships.

Look at your 'life sentences'

Now think about the internal sentences that run in your head and can run you and the life you live. These 'life sentences' are based on your experiences of relationships, and your self-esteem; as the Jesuits say, *'Give me a child until he is seven and I will give you the man.'*

Messages from authority figures can be implanted deep within you in childhood and can be very powerful; they can make you or break you. We are, after all, dependent on others for many years. Good parents are purposefully shaping their children's brains for a long time, getting them ready to be self-regulating adults. So, no wonder sources of authority – parents and their substitutes, like teachers – can have such a profound effect. With adolescence comes the start of testing the system against peer pressures – a kind of first run at trying to be grown up.

We all have sentences running in our heads that were created in childhood and continue to be triggered throughout life. Perhaps your mother never told you that you were pretty, or your father repeatedly said you were stupid or too fat? Perhaps your teacher said there was no point in taking exams because 'you would never pass'? These experiences, often said casually, can paralyse you in different ways – although it is also true that sometimes they can be the spur to proving someone else completely wrong.

We store these life sentences and incorporate them into our narrative; they are the scripts by which we live. Our brains make sense of negative experiences and their emotional turbulence by awarding them the status of a higher truth and build stories off the back of them. These stories go on to inform the beliefs we hold about who we are, what we are and are not capable of, and what we are responsible for.

We can also give 'life sentences' to ourselves, often inappropriately. For example, children whose parents divorced often carry the burden of feeling that somehow, they themselves were responsible for it and should have been able to do something about it. We can also make early life decisions that are hugely beneficial. Many individuals who become doctors or research scientists can recall the childhood moment when they made the decision that's what they wanted to 'be'. Negative – and positive – self-beliefs can develop as a consequence of your role within your family. You may have been labelled as the 'scatty', 'clever', 'lucky' or 'slow' one, and it's possible to spend decades of life living up (or down) to the role ascribed to you.

Do you never try anything because 'you will never pass'? Do you never comment at work or with friends and never put yourself forward, because 'you are stupid'? Some people even turn to alcohol, drugs or overeating to dull this pain. The words of a life sentence become your destiny unless and until you recognise why they are there, and, from your adult standpoint, realise that you can free yourself from these inner demons.

Using your notebook, identify, and write down, any 'sentences' that are ruling your life. Again, quiet your mind, sit still and ask for them to come into your head. Can you remember where they came from? Who said them and why? Once you recognise what is running you, it is very much easier to free yourself from it.

If you are not sure where to start look at these examples:

I never...	I always...
My life is...	I am stupid...
I will never be a success...	No one loves me...
I don't love anyone...	I am afraid...
I don't need anyone...	I am not trustworthy...
I am not good enough...	I am not pretty...
Partners always leave me...	I will never have money...
I am always ill...	I never get better...
No one is ever there for me...	I am always on my own...
People don't like me...	I always feel tired...
I am always being criticised...	I can never decide...
I am always stressed...	I never have time...

Are you emotionally 'stuck'?

Can you express your feelings easily, or do you experience life more placidly? Emotions range from one extreme to another – from delirious joy to suicidal despair, from trust and love through to rage, anger and jealousy. Ideally, you should be able to dip in and out of all of them, even into difficult emotions like terror, rage or hopelessness, at appropriate times, if only for a few moments or even seconds.

Traumatic events in the past, or the behaviours of difficult people, often cause us, subliminally, or non-consciously, to block off feelings that we have judged 'not for us'. This is usually a self-protection mechanism, set up because the way they made us feel seemed so difficult to deal with. But these blocks are rarely helpful in the long term. They may have been useful at the time, but keeping them in place for life can create other problems.

For example, people who grew up terrified by angry, shouting fathers, can sometimes block rage and anger as emotional responses. This is because, first, it shielded them from further abuse and, secondly, they refuse to repeat the same pattern in their own lives. As adults, however, if you never let yourself become angry, you may struggle with not being heard, never speaking up or perceiving yourself as being weak. You may not dare to negotiate your own interests effectively, or to risk interpersonal conflict even when the outcome could be productive.

It is all about balance. Balance in the regulating of emotions is one of the keys to a healthy life. Think harmony, like the playing of a piano: there may be loud and soft passages in a piece of music, but overall they balance each other because the whole system is well regulated. So it is with emotions. Most of us feel comfortable with the 'safe' middle-range emotions, but it is also possible to enjoy strong emotions when they are appropriate and well regulated. It's a question of not letting yourself be overwhelmed by any extreme feeling, and not shutting yourself off entirely from any emotion. Expressing yourself, with an unfamiliar emotion, even for a few seconds, can be liberating and help you to change your life.

Bach flower remedies

Discovered by Dr Edward Bach in the early 20th century, these 38 remedies can help you to release difficult to deal with mind states and relieve specific emotions. Add a few drops of your chosen remedy to a 30ml bottle of water and take four drops four times a day. There is even a Rescue remedy for emergency stress relief which contains a combination of five essences.

Agrimony for mental torture behind a cheerful face

continued...

Aspen for fear of unknown things

Beech for intolerance

Centaury for the inability to say 'no'

Cerato for lack of trust in one's own decisions

Cherry plum for fear of the mind giving way

Chestnut bud for failure to learn from mistakes

Chicory for selfish, possessive love

Clematis for dreaming of the future without working in the present

Crab apple for the cleansing remedy, also for self-hatred

Elm for overwhelmed by responsibility

Gentian for discouragement after a setback

Gorse for hopelessness and despair

Heather for self-centredness and self-concern

Holly for hatred, envy and jealousy

Honeysuckle for living in the past

Hornbeam for tiredness at the thought of doing something

Impatiens for impatience

Larch for lack of confidence

Mimulus for fear of known things

Mustard for deep gloom for no reason

Oak for the plodder who keeps going past the point of exhaustion

Olive for exhaustion following mental or physical effort

Pine for guilt

Red chestnut for over-concern for the welfare of loved ones

Rock rose for terror and fright

Rock water for self-denial, rigidity and self-repression

Scleranthus for inability to choose between alternatives

Star of Bethlehem for shock

Sweet chestnut for extreme mental anguish, when everything has been tried and there is no light left

Vervain for over-enthusiasm

continued...

Vine for dominance and inflexibility

Walnut for protection from change and unwanted influences

Water violet for quiet self-reliance leading to isolation

White chestnut for unwanted thoughts and mental arguments

Wild oat for uncertainty over one's direction in life

Wild rose for drifting, resignation, apathy

Willow for self-pity and resentment

The eight basic emotions

Our emotions control our behaviour and make sense of the world for us. Experience is first attached to emotion and then distributed into feelings (which also generate moods and states). The psychologist Antonio Damasio uses the analogy of thinking about the basic emotions as if they were primary colours. So, just as the whole of the colour palette comes from a base of three primary colours, so the whole of the feeling spectrum stems similarly from the eight basic emotions: sadness, shame, disgust, anger, fear, surprise or startle, excitement or joy, love or trust. Links

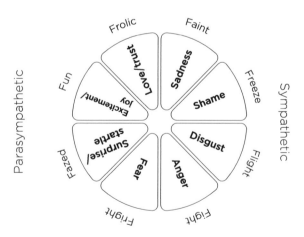

have been identified between the emotions and the autonomic nervous system. The sympathetic and parasympathetic systems react to specific feelings. Anger, for example, instantly triggers a fight response, and fear, a fright reaction.

Did you know... Emotions trigger reactions?

'There is nothing either good or bad,
but thinking makes it so...'

WILLIAM SHAKESPEARE, HAMLET

Emotions are the triggers for every action we take. You may believe that your actions occur as a result of your thoughts, but science now shows us otherwise. In reality, first you experience an emotion attached to an experience to which you give a certain meaning and only then, as a consequence of that emotion, consciously or non-consciously, do you take action. All in a split second of time.

Emotions organise how your brain works and thinks, and are closely tied into your autonomic nervous system – automatically and functioning at a deep and non-conscious level. Your nervous system has two branches – the sympathetic nervous system, which is geared for survival – flight, fight, flight, freeze/faint – and the parallel and balancing parasympathetic nervous system – home of excitement, joy and trust, and love.

The brain can organise itself for action in 85 milliseconds, yet awareness doesn't kick in until 250 milliseconds. So the truth is that your brain is in charge of you – rather than, as you might have thought, you in charge of your brain, but, ultimately, it is emotion that rules the brain, and 'you'.[13]

Exercise: What emotions can you feel?

Again, sit quietly with your notepad, and see if you can identify any patterns in your emotional behaviour. The names we give the emotions are a way of making sense of what the body is experiencing. Think about which emotions you are not comfortable with, or which ones you can't feel and why? Look at each one. If you judge it as unacceptable, do you remember why?

Which emotions do you find hardest to regulate? Try to identify the original memory that caused the problem from your list of past stressors. It may relate to a few, separate memories that set in your mind a particular, negative view of yourself. It may be that the emotion in question was not part of the emotional currency in your family so you are not familiar with it – as if using it felt much like trying a foreign language.

Now think about where you feel the stronger emotions in your body. Make a note of what that sensation is like. Is it a flutter in your throat, a stabbing pain in your stomach or a warmth in your heart? Once you have registered where that sensation shows up, and how, and can make the connection with the emotion associated with it, you can consciously choose to adjust your behaviour or feelings in the future. Awareness is halfway to healing.

Change your mind: Re-write your life

'Declutter your brain, release yesterday's stresses, and your today will flow more smoothly. Science proves it.'

Sara Davenport

The next challenge is to rewrite your internal script. Here's an exercise that can help you do this – if you really want to that is...

Exercise: How to discard unhelpful beliefs

Taking the events on your life stress list, above, and your unhelpful beliefs, one at a time, allow yourself to really feel them – for example, the belief 'I'm stupid', might lead to feelings of shame and worthlessness. Let yourself sit with each feeling and acknowledge how it affects your body. Does it manifest as an unsettled feeling deep in the pit of your stomach, or oppressive tension in your chest? You may find that old memories related to the feeling surface, too: make a note of these.

First, feel the memory

When a difficult event happens, people are often so caught up in the sheer speed of the event that the feelings that came with it had no time to be felt or even acknowledged. Usually they bury them deep, meaning to return to them at a later date when everything has passed, but never actually getting around to it. The feelings sit in the closed cupboards of your psyche, behind doors you would much rather not open – however, your non-conscious mind also knows that the 'stuff' inside needs to be not only acknowledged, but released. A constant battle wages between the part of you that would prefer not to look, and the part that wants to be free.

The most important part of this exercise is to then magnify the feeling. The frequency of an emotion is very similar to the frequency of sound: intensity is the key. Rather like the opera singer whose party trick is to sing a single note at a champagne glass, higher and higher, until the glass shatters, a low intensity of feeling won't shift an emotion – or release an event – that has been running you for years. But if you let yourself feel that emotion very deeply, even just for a second or two, the intensity of the feeling effectively releases the hold it has had over you. Your non-conscious mind can finally let go and relax – because, instead of yet again avoiding the issue and burying it again, you have finally examined it and truly felt the emotions that were by-passed at the time. This releases any blockage in the mental energy field created at the time, much in the same way as clearing a blockage of twigs and debris in a stream allows the water to run freely once again. The feeling can now be put back in your 'library' of memories and pulled out at will, without any 'charge' attached to it; your non-conscious mind no longer needs to keep bringing it to the forefront of your mind.

Now set yourself free

To set yourself free from a painful memory, you need to acquire the power that was taken from you, or believed you did not have – and so were not able to exercise – when you were dumped by your partner, your teacher criticised you publicly, or your schoolmates jeered at you.

It is possible to release the past in a very private and simple way by re-imagining what happened. Your mind always holds onto the last 'recorded' image of anything that happens. So, you simply need to imprint another ending. Visualise the original event in your mind's eye, but insert a very different outcome into the memory, in whatever way feels appropriate to you. It's a bit like the relief you feel in your shoulders when you take off a heavy rucksack. You'll feel a similar sense of relief as you change the script of that painful 'mind movie'. You might have an imaginary argument inside your head with the unkind ex-partner or harsh parent who sowed the seed of negativity – tell them 'That's not true,' or shout 'Rubbish!' at them. Or you might see the word, written in giant letters, 'FAT', or 'SELFISH', or whatever it might be, then imagine yourself knocking the enormous foam letters down with a stick, stamping on them, or even setting fire to them. The more creative, vivid and 'out-there' the visualisation, the more memorable and helpful it will be.

How does it work?

From your brain's point of view, what you are doing is attaching new chemicals – and hence new emotions – to old events. As I have already mentioned, your brain will do its best to hold on to the old stuff – just in case the 'life sentence' is true – after all, it kept you safe all these years. So, even when you feel you really have said goodbye to it, there may be occasions when up it pops again, for example, if your immune system is low and you are feeling weak, perhaps with a virus, as the energy needed to keep the 'new' in place has been diverted to fight the infection. The more deeply entrenched your new emotions become, however, the less that will happen. And as a result of your new awareness, you will be able to recognise them when they arise and so put them back in the new place – you have begun the process of permanently altering them.

Once you trust yourself to recognise the unhelpful labels you have been unknowingly pinning on yourself, you can laugh at them, or shout down the disparaging voice in your head, using the re-framing visualisations you created to dismantle the apparatus of self-criticism. Over time, this will allow the space and confidence for a healthier, more accurate and kinder internal script to develop.

It is remarkable that visualisation and imagining something happening in advance really does create new pathways in the brain and make new connections to old experience. But so it is, and these exercises will let you make the most of this amazing ability. But you do need to actually generate the new emotions; just thinking of them won't work, it's *experiencing* them that counts.

Re-create your mental landscape

Focused intention is key to 're-structuring' your brain, both emotionally and physically. Now it's time to move forward and specify your intentions precisely, find your purpose, and make greater connections. The exercises here will help you to do this.

> ## Did you know...?
> People who have a sense of purpose have been shown to be happier than those that don't.[14] They sleep better, are less likely to develop depression or other mental health problems, or dementia, and live longer.[15]

Exercise 1: Learn to focus your intention

It's crucial to define your intentions for yourself and they need to be precise. Your non-conscious mind interprets intentions as 'orders' and will carry them out as given if you set them up as instructions – it doesn't work if you only set them up as 'hopes', or 'likes'. For example, 'Yes, I would like to be the person I think I could be' just won't get you there. The brain knows it's a hypothesis – it's rather like saying where you would like to go on holiday without doing anything about it.

Sit down quietly and internally give the specific orders that will establish you as the best that you can imagine being. You need to make a shift in how you think about yourself. For example, 'I'd like to stop smoking', won't work. But saying, 'I will work out what a non-smoker does, and do that', will. Non-smokers, for instance, don't buy cigarettes. This is not because they have told themselves not to buy them, but because, being non-smokers, they simply don't.

See yourself becoming 'you'. The non-conscious mind reads pictures better than words, so use imagery and visualisation to create the results you want. Always imagine a scene in the present because for the non-conscious mind, there is only the now and it only responds to 'present-moment' instructions. And always see the image you are working on as a positive. Your non-conscious mind will ignore anything pictured in the past or the future – even though, of course, the present can only be construed in terms of the past which, being the past, is the only past you could have had whatever else you might retrospectively wish. And there is nothing to be gained by telling yourself what you *don't* want to be either. That's like telling yourself where you don't want to go on holiday; you would never book flights there or look forward to the experience.

Do this exercise regularly, several times a day. Your brain gets convinced by practice – just like learning a new language. New pathways need creating and then strengthening and then they become habits. Always rehearse the positive – if you rehearse the negative, all you will get is negative. Focus on exhaustion or being slow or stupid, and your brain will deliver that image. See yourself mentally as whatever it is you intend to be, however, and your brain will work to deliver you that image instead. Picture the final result right from the start. Always see yourself right now, and focus very specifically on seeing your new improved, modified Self as the 'you' with whom you are pleased.

Exercise 2: Find your purpose

Purpose is what gives meaning to your existence. Without some sense of purpose your brain may struggle with a weight of exhaustion that you may be unaware of – for example, do you find it hard to get up in the morning with no particular focus to your day?

A purpose doesn't have to be a grand global statement, it's just about something that is important in your life and there is no wrong or right to it. It is simply something that makes your heart sing, is worthwhile and, as a result of doing it, life feels 'worth it'. It could be to bring up healthy, happy children, to love animals, to become a florist or retrain as an accountant. It could be knowing that you brighten the life of the old lady down the road by visiting her once a week, or the pleasure you get from digging the garden every day, or singing in a choir.

In 2014, when asked about the meaning of life, the Dalai Lama simply replied, 'happiness'. What happiness is for you, only you know. Find a purpose for living and your mind will rally. But happiness is an outcome, not something to be pursued for its own sake. The wise, long-exiled Vietnamese monk Thich Nhat Hanh once said: *'There is no way to happiness. Happiness is the way.'*[16]

Sit down somewhere quiet, and think about what you would really like to do – for yourself. This is not about being sensible or making money, but what would bring you joy. It might be something you haven't done for years or something you have always dreamt of doing, but somehow never got around to. Write a list, and then pick. You will be well on your way to finding your purpose.

Exercise 3: Make a connection to something greater than yourself

There are many different names for that invisible power – spirit, energy, love, higher self, God. Studies show that people who have a spiritual practice of some kind are happier. Read spiritual writings, meditate, say a daily personal prayer, or give thanks for the good things in your life. It doesn't have to be a religious practice and they don't have to be religious books, though they can be. Read about love, compassion and gratitude, and incorporate those qualities into your daily life. Just the act of turning your attention to those thoughts and feelings increases your spiritual strength. It can be a huge relief to discover that there is something else in the Universe guiding and sustaining you and you can hand over control of what often seems a rocky ride in life.

Brain entrainment

Think carefully about the company you keep, whether at home, amongst friends, or with work colleagues. You really do pick up emotions from those around you. Science has shown that emotions, just like diseases, are contagious; fear and anger are as equally easy to take on board as joy and contentment. The radiator and drain analogy now has science to back it: negative associates really do drain your energy, and likewise, positive, life-affirming friends, really do boost your energy field. Your brain aligns itself with those you keep in close contact with and entrains your energy field with theirs. Whatever your own frequency you will attract others tuned to the same bandwidth.[17]

STEP TWO

—

REPAIR
your
Brain

'What you do today can improve all your tomorrows.'

RALPH MARSTON, MOTIVATOR AND COACH

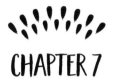

CHAPTER 7

ACTION! WHAT TO EAT AND HOW TO MOVE

*'You can make your brain better, even if you've
been bad to it...'*

Daniel G Amen MD

A ll sorts of things impact your brain, but what you eat and how much you exercise are right up there. Both support brain function from the outset, but in some situations they might prevent, and even counteract, cognitive decline.

First, I've compiled some dietary recommendations based around the foods that have been shown to improve brain function. Then I've done the same with exercise. The importance of exercise for brain health has hit the headlines again, with evidence to support the fact that cardiovascular exercise is one of the most effective ways to boost neuroplasticity. For most of us, the issue is finding time and energy to work out enough, but, for a super-fit minority, the balance may need to tip in the opposite direction to optimise brain health. With exercise, too much of a good thing can have a net-negative impact on cognitive function, so it's important to get the balance right. More of that later, though.

What to Eat

The food you choose to eat has a huge impact on your brain. According to Drs Dean and Ayesha Sherzai at Loma Linda University, California, USA, more than 90 per cent of Alzheimer's cases can be prevented with simple lifestyle and dietary changes. Thanks to an overwhelming increase in scientific interest in the relationship between nutrition and the brain, we now know more than ever before about the way food can support – or sabotage – healthy brain function.[1] The problem is that much of this information appears contradictory, and many of the most important insights are buried in dense scientific studies that only the most dedicated researcher has the time to sift through. So, I have done the work for you.

General dietary advice

There is a long list of specific foods that have known brain-benefits. But look at the bigger picture first – how should you approach your diet? Stable blood sugar supports optimal brain function, so, as a general rule, a low glycaemic load (LGL) diet, avoiding refined carbohydrates and sugary foods, is a great place to start. Increasing your intake of plant-based wholefoods is also a good idea – plenty of fruit and vegetables and unprocessed wholegrains will ensure your brain has the nutrients it needs to flourish. For those who eat fish, omega-3 rich oily fish is a good addition; eat it once or twice a week. If you are vegetarian or vegan, there are other sources of essential fatty acids, for example, chia seeds, hemp and nuts, and cold-pressed nut oils. Avocado and eggs are good brain foods too. But, before we get into the specifics of what to eat, a word on pesticides.

Should you eat organic foods?

I do recommend buying organic whenever you can, and can afford to. I'm aware, however, that most research appears to show that organic food isn't demonstrably more nutritious. A 2009 meta-analysis found there was no nutrient difference between organic and non-organic food,[2] and similar studies have found only a minimal difference. Milk, however, appears to be an exception. Not only does organic milk contain more omega-3 fatty acid, but there are studies showing that it has a higher antioxidant count.

The nutrients are one thing, but the extra, unwanted consumption of pesticides and fungicides is another. Reducing your consumption of synthetic pesticides and fungicides is likely to be good news for your brain health. Many studies that looked at the impact of pesticides on farm workers' children (whose mothers worked in the fields during pregnancy) found that the greater the mother's exposure to pesticides, the higher the likelihood of neurological problems and cognitive impairment in their children.[3] Although these mothers (and therefore developing foetuses) were exposed to far higher levels of pesticide than you or I would be when consuming the sprayed produce, it seems logical to infer that a lower-level, but similar impact on the brain could result from consuming produce that contains high levels of pesticides.

Studies show a mind-boggling variety of pesticide traces on conventionally farmed produce. One recent American study (where farmers are allowed to use a number of pesticides banned in the European Union/EU) found that multiple kale samples had traces of 18 pesticides, even after they had been washed.[4] In light of this, it's perhaps not surprising that the overwhelming majority of consumers who buy organic cite environmental impact as their main motivator, with concern over pesticides at the top of the list.[5] There is growing awareness of the potential impact of pesticides on brain function, and in 2017 an EU panel of experts concluded that organic produce was likely to pose less of a threat to brain health.

A word of caution, though. It's important to remember that organic doesn't mean pesticide-free. It's just that any pesticides used must be naturally derived and there are fewer of them. When something is 'natural' it always sounds safe, but some of these 'natural' pesticides can be just as bad for you, and/or even be worse for the environment than their synthetic counterparts. What's more, pesticides such as rotenone, occasionally used in organic farming in the UK as a 'last resort', have been linked to the development of Parkinson's disease in the farm workers who administer it.[6] All this makes our choice as consumers feel fraught with risk.

What then is the solution, if you don't have the time, space or inclination to grow your own? So, rather than thinking organic vs. non-organic, I recommend you consider a middle road. Minimise the foods that are most likely to be farmed with heavy pesticide use, such as citrus fruits, strawberries, lettuce, pears and grapes. Buy organic whenever you can and wash everything (organic and non-organic) thoroughly. There's an interesting product called 'sonic soak' that uses ultrasonic wave technology to deep-clean vegetables and fruit. You simply put the device in a bowl of water with your vegetables and it cleans them of pesticides (and dirt and bacteria).

Some foods also contain more pesticide residue than others so I'd also recommend increasing your intake of the foods on the table opposite as they are the ones found by UK studies done between 2011 and 2015[7] to have the lowest pesticide residues.

Ranking	Produce	Single residue occurrence %	Multiple residue occurrence %
1	Beetroot	7.41	0
2	Cauliflower	0.00	0
3	Corn (on the cob)	0.00	0
4	Figs	4.17	0
5	Mushrooms	33.33	0
6	Onions	70.83	0
7	Rhubarb	2.44	0
8	Swede	14.00	0
9	Turnip	0.00	0
10	Peas	11.46	1.04
11	Spring onions	25.00	1.39
12	Asparagus	8.33	2.08
13	Radish	53.70	3.7
14	Avocado	44.44	4.44
15	Peas without pods	23.96	5.21
16	Sweet potato	58.33	5.56
17	Leeks	15.63	6.25
18	Broad Beans	43.75	8.33
19	Pumpkin and Squash	31.25	8.33
20	Broccoli	25.60	9.52

My father's brain diet

In addition to the lower-pesticide-residue foods listed in the box above, there are a number of other foods that have been proven to have a specific brain-health benefit. Based on the science, these are the foods we introduced into my father's diet. It is not an exhaustive list of beneficial foods, but it serves as a good guide to what can make a difference to your brain function.

Wholegrain foods

Our ability to sustain concentration relies on stable blood sugar levels – fluctuations caused by disproportionate lows following high-sugar snacks or meals, can lead to irritability and loss of concentration. Wholegrains are also packed with other nutrients, including the B-vitamins and fibre. Switching white pasta and bread to wholegrain varieties will also have a beneficial impact on the bacterial flora in your gut, which is likely to benefit your brain function. Be adventurous with wholegrains, too – try unrefined grains such as quinoa, black rice, spelt and freekeh.

Fruit and vegetables

Blueberries and raspberries (and other dark red and purple fruit and vegetables) A review of studies by researchers at Tufts University, Massachusets, USA, concluded that berry fruits protect brain cells from damage and prevent inflammation.[8] They found a correlation between berry consumption and a reduced risk of Alzheimer's disease, which they believe is down to the anthocyanins, or antioxidant flavonoids, that give them their colour. These antioxidants help fight oxidative stress. Raspberries in particular are a great choice as they contain notably low levels of sugar compared with other fruits. I recommend buying organic berries, but, as I mentioned earlier, the jury is still out, and non-organic is unquestionably better than nothing.

Tomatoes These fruits are packed with lycopene, a powerful antioxidant that becomes more bio-available when it's cooked. Lycopene can help protect against free-radical cell damage, the type that occurs in dementia, and particularly in Alzheimer's disease.

Broccoli This everyday superfood is rich in vitamin K, a key nutrient for supporting cognitive function and brain power. Broccoli also contains high levels of glucosinolates, which help to slow the breakdown of a key neurotransmitter, acetylcholine. The degeneration of acetylcholine has been associated with neurodegenerative diseases, so upping your broccoli intake could also be a good way to protect yourself.[9]

Leafy dark green vegetables These are an excellent source of folate (the natural form of vitamin B9) as well as other vitamins, and minerals such as copper and fibre.

Spices

Cinnamon Shown to reduce inflammation and oxidation in the brain, cinnamon improves memory in people with learning difficulties and, in studies on mice, has been found to protect dopamine production and improve motor function in people with Parkinson's disease.[10] It has a positive effect on the hippocampus area of the brain and may protect against Alzheimer's disease.

Turmeric This commonly used spice has been the subject of a huge number of studies focused on its neuroprotective benefits. It is thought to be the main reason why curry consumption appears to protect against cognitive decline. Studies on elderly Asians show that curcumin, the active ingredient in turmeric, appears to be able to cross the blood–brain barrier, and reduce the effects of brain inflammation, boosting memory. A supplement made by PuraTHRIVE, micelle curcumin, which has curcumin suspended in ginger oil and vegan DHA, increases bioavailability of the curcuminoids in turmeric 185 times.

Legumes

Chickpeas, lentils, brown or white beans, and peas contain iron, magnesium, potassium and folate (the natural form of vitamin B9 found in foods; folic acid is the synthetic form) that help boost the firing of your brain neurons. Legumes also contain choline, which boosts the neurotransmitter acetylcholine vital for brain health.

Nuts and seeds

Nuts slow down the ageing of the brain. They are packed with vitamin E, a nutrient that has been shown to be protective against cognitive decline, particularly in the elderly.[11] They also contain essential fatty acids. Research carried out at Loma Linda University, California, USA, showed that pistachios had the most beneficial impact on memory of all the nuts.

Pumpkin seeds All seeds are good for you, but pumpkin seeds are particularly high in zinc, a vital mineral that has been found to support memory and clear thinking. Pumpkin seeds are also packed with magnesium, which calms the mind, and contain the all-important B vitamins, as well as L-tryptophan, the amino acid that helps your body produce the 'happy hormone', serotonin.

Coconut oil

Although it's important not to overdo it with coconut oil because it's high in saturated fat, eating a small amount regularly could improve brain function. Studies into the potential neuroprotective benefit of coconut oil are ongoing, with some indications that coconut oil may help reduce and reverse the neurodegenerative effects characteristic of dementia.[12]

Omega-3-rich foods

A range of studies show that eating and supplementation with omega-3's boosts a number of aspects of cognitive function.[13]

Oily fish This is an excellent source of omega-3 fatty acids. Opt for wild salmon, rather than farmed, as it tends to be leaner. Smaller fish such as sardines, anchovies and mackerel are good too. However, concern over mercury levels (particularly high in large species such as tuna, but also present in smaller species such as sardines and anchovies) may put you off.

Plant-based omega-3s For those who would prefer to avoid fish, there are plant-based sources of omega-3 rich alternatives such as flax, hemp, chia seed, and seaweed.

Green tea

This is packed with antioxidants known to support neuroplasticity. L-Theanine, the active ingredient in green tea, has been found to reduce cortisol levels and increase BDNF (brain-derived neurotrophic factor), the protein that promotes neuroplasticity.[14]

Coffee

Caffeine makes you feel more alert, and some studies have linked consumption with improved memory. Up to four cups of coffee a day has been found to incrementally boost focus and memory recall.[15] In older adults, coffee consumption is correlated with reduced rates of cognitive decline. Coffee is also good for your reaction time, memory, and overall cognitive function. The benefits are thought to be a result of the way caffeine blocks your adenosine receptors, preventing the release of excitatory brain chemicals. With this blocked, you get a surge of brain energy. Coffee expands the blood vessels that feed the brain, so helping circulation. Drink it black to maximise the benefits as adding milk decreases the antioxidant activity of the polyphenols. Avoid caffeine after midday, though, as it can affect sleep, see Chapter 9.

Pure dark chocolate

The flavonoids found in pure dark chocolate (and it must be pure) create angiogenesis, neurogenesis and changes in neuron morphology, mainly in brain regions involved in learning and memory.[16] Epicatechin, for example, improves various aspects of cognition in animals and humans. Chocolate also induces positive effects on mood and is often consumed under emotional stress. It also contains phenylethylamine (PEA), which encourages the brain to release pleasure-enhancing endorphins that relieve depression and anxiety and boost feelings of wellbeing.[17] In addition, flavonoids have been seen to preserve cognitive abilities during ageing in rats, and lower the risk of developing Alzheimer's disease and decrease the risk of stroke in humans.[18]

Eggs

Although moderation is key with eggs, due to their high cholesterol and fat content, they are a great source of vitamin B12 and folate (B9). Both vitamins reduce levels of homocysteine in the blood; a high level of homocysteine is associated with increased risk of stroke, cognitive impairment and Alzheimer's disease. In an American study, elderly adults showing signs of cognitive impairment saw some of their symptoms reversed after two years of B vitamin supplementation.[19] If you don't eat eggs, you can get the same benefit from eating chicken, fish or leafy green vegetables. Vegans will need to supplement with B12 to get the required amount.

Fermented foods

Kimchi, sauerkraut, and some pickles, although often loaded with salt, are great for your gut bacteria, as is kefir, which can be fermented from either cow or goat milk. These foods contain the probiotic bacteria *lactobacillus plantarum* (see page 267 for more on this), a probiotic bacteria that has a stress-lowering response.

Consider intermittent fasting

There's been a lot of press coverage recently around the benefits of intermittent fasting, with Silicon Valley heavyweights like Jeff Bezos going on the record about the virtues of on–off eating. I was sceptical at first, but there is credible evidence to suggest that calorie restriction and fasting can increase neuroplasticity, which promotes neuron growth and reduces inflammation. The metabolic shift that results also lowers levels of leptin in the body, which sends a chemical signal instructing the neurons to produce more energy. The net effect is improved cognitive function.[20]

There are a number of ways to try it. Some are more demanding than others. Popular methods include fasting for 24 hours (once a week). More do-able is a scaled-back version – a 16-hour fast, so you might eat your evening meal at 6pm one night, then not eat again until 10am the following day. There is also the 5–2 model, where you have five days of regular eating, and two (non-consecutive) days of calorie-restricted eating in a week.

Supplements that boost your brain

There are a number of vitamins, minerals and other supplements that can have a specific effect on the brain. You may have come across the buzzword 'nootropics' either in the supplements section of your health food shop or you might have read about them. Nootropics are 'cognitive enhancers', or substances that are proven to improve a range of aspects of mental function, including memory, intelligence, motivation, attention and concentration, while doing no harm. Some are single-source supplements, such as omega-3s from fish oil or gingko biloba, but many comprise a combination of ingredients and nutrients. The compound supplements tend to contain a mixture of essential fatty acids, amino acids and other nutrients.

Some nootropic combination supplements have a sound evidence-base behind them, and you'll save time, hassle and money in the long run by buying them, but for the purposes of clarity, I think it's worth running through individual nutrients one by one to outline their brain-boosting benefits and the evidence that backs it up. That way, you can assess the individual components and work out which nutrients are most likely to be beneficial to you. I have presented them in A to Z order, but you need to check the labels of the compound supplements and work out which contain the nutrients you need.

Acetyl-l-carnitine

This is an amino acid that plays an important role in cell metabolism and delivers essential fatty acids to your cells, where they can be metabolised. A 2010 study found that acetyl-l-carnitine improved learning capacity in ageing rats,[21] and it is recommended as an anti-ageing brain supplement,[22] marketed as a way to boost 'brain energy'. Two Italian research trials at

Catania University, reported improvements in cognitive function in adults with fatigue.[23] However, no conclusive evidence on the benefits for dementia patients has been published.

Alpha glycerophosphocholine (alpha-GPC)

A chemical released when a fatty acid found in soya and other plants breaks down, alpha-GPC, contains choline and appears to raise levels of the neurotransmitter acetylcholine and possibly dopamine in the brain. In some European countries it is prescribed to people with dementia and those who have suffered a stroke; in the USA it is only available as a supplement.

Alpha lipoic acid (ALA)

This compound, found in mitochondria and produced by the body in small quantities, has been found to strongly protect the brain from oxidative damage. It has been seen to stimulate brain cell growth and aid brain recovery after a stroke in rats.[24] It is also a powerful anti-inflammatory,[25] significant in the brain as inflammation is known to cause neurodegenerative symptoms.

Amino acids, especially creatine and taurine

Creatine Found abundantly in 'muscle meat', particularly red meat and pork, creatine is most often associated with body-building. But a 2018 review of six randomised controlled trials on the impact of creatine supplementation on brain function caught my attention.[26] The review found that short-term memory and reasoning appeared to be enhanced across the board by supplementation, although evidence for other improvements (in executive function, reaction time and mental fatigue) were more conflicted. A range of creatine supplements are available, many from whey-based (milk) sources, although you can also buy synthetic creatine.

Taurine Debate is ongoing about whether this amino acid should be categorised as a neurotransmitter, as it structurally and functionally resembles one.[27] It has been found to play a key role in the survival and growth of neurons as it shares a receptor with gama aminobutyric acid or GABA (the brain's foremost inhibitory neurotransmitter, which has a calming influence in the brain), and scientists are still working to understand its function.[28]

Astaxanthin

An antioxidant that can cross both the blood–brain and blood–retinal barriers, and so reach all the cells in your brain, astaxanthin reduces oxidative damage by protecting mitochondria and neurons from free radicals. It is thought to boost production of neural stem cells. It improves memory and slows inflammation.

Bacopa monnieri (BM)

An Ayurvedic herbal remedy, BM, also known as brahmi, is often recommended as an anti-Alzheimer's and anti-anxiety remedy, and there is evidence to back up both claims. Until relatively recently, studies have been animal-based, but a 2001 trial on adults, focusing on memory recall, found a significant association between bacopa supplementation and reduced memory loss over a three-month period.[29] A 2013 review examined the findings and concluded that several randomised, double-blind, placebo-controlled trials substantiated BM's nootropic utility in humans. There is also evidence for potential reduction in symptoms of dementia, Parkinson's disease, and epilepsy.[30] BM's nootropic benefits are due to its antioxidant activity. BM also appears to increase brain–blood flow and help modulate neurotransmitters.

Cannabis

Cannabis affects the brain positively in regard to memory, mood and cognition. It releases the feel-good neurotransmitters such as such as dopamine and serotonin. Different forms of cannabis affect different parts of the brain and areas of function. (See reference section pages 270-72 for more information).

Citicoline (CDP-Choline)

A synthetic substance that mimics a natural substance with neuroprotective benefits, citicoline, or CDP-choline, is a popular ingredient in brain-boosting supplements. Choline is a vitamin-like nutrient that has become something of a nootropic buzzword. A 2014 paper authored by Professor Pawel Grieb, analysed a wide range of clinical trials and concluded that: *'There is no adequate description of the mechanism(s) of the pharmacological actions of this substance.'* As such, its beneficial activity is hard to define and measure, although the trial data appeared to show the most benefit in slow-advancing neurodegenerative disorders.[31]

Copper

Like iron, below, this trace element performs a key role in brain function. The correct amount and metabolism of copper is essential to maintain the ideal biochemistry of the brain to support the production of neurotransmitters. Excessive copper has been linked to neurodegenerative disorder,[32] so the key is balance.[33] Copper deficiency can result from gastrointestinal surgery or gastric disorders, and has implications for heart health.[34] The best dietary sources are nuts, seeds, leafy green vegetables, pure dark chocolate, oysters and shitake mushrooms.

CoQ10

Supplementing with CoQ10 can increase the size of the cerebral cortex (see page 19) and boost mitochondrial strength, so protecting against neurodegenerative disease and reducing oxidation.[35]

Curcumin

An extract of turmeric root, which gives turmeric its distinctive colour and flavour (most ground turmeric contains only 3–4 per cent curcumin[36]), curcumin has been found to have powerful anti-inflammatory benefits. A University of California study focused on 40 older adults who were complaining of memory lapses, but did not have symptoms of dementia. After twice-daily supplementation with 80mg of a high-potency curcumin extract, theracumin, significant improvements in memory, attention and mood were observed.[37] Look for AlphaCurcuminPlus, which contains phospholipids so that the curcumin is absorbed many times faster than from other products.

Gingko

Often recommended by herbalists as a supplement to help ward off cognitive impairment, gingko, from the gingko biloba tree, has also been marketed as a memory booster. Large-scale clinical trial evidence is patchy, although a 2010 European study found a significant delay in the onset of Alzheimer's symptoms in patients who had supplemented with gingko for four years, when compared to a control group.[38]

Glutathione

A powerful antioxidant, glutathione in liposomal form protects against cognitive impairment, lowering inflammation levels and neutralising oxidative stress.[39] Conversely, it has been found that people suffering from depression and anxiety, autism, schizophrenia, bi-polar disorder and obsessive compulsive disorder (OCD) have lower than normal levels of glutathione.

Gotu kola

This is a traditional Chinese, Indonesian, and Ayurvedic herbal remedy, whose Chinese name means 'fountain of youth'. Gotu kola is believed to extend life and boost brain function. In studies, it reduced depression and anxiety by 50 per cent and increased mental alertness by 100 per cent.[40]

Huperzine A

Recognised for its 'neuroprotective' qualities this extract (which derives from certain club fir-moss plants) is also used in some drug treatments for Alzheimer's disease. There has been some debate in the USA as to whether it should not be sold as a food 'supplement', but classified as a drug instead. A 2014 review found that it not only improved memory and protected nerve cells in people with dementia, but could slow down the cognitive decline associated with Alzheimer's disease.[41] Huperzine A appears to play a part in regulating nerve growth factor in the brain (reduced nerve growth has been observed in people with Alzheimer's), and a 2013 meta-analysis of studies found that memory scores improved after supplementation.[42]

Iron

This is a mineral essential to healthy brain function. It plays a role in offsetting oxidative stress, and is a co-factor in the synthesis of certain neurotransmitters and myelin[43] – the fatty substance that insulates neuronal activity (the speed, connectivity and efficiency of the pathways in the brain) and a key aspect of neuroplasticity. There are two forms of iron – heme iron (the type found in meat, and the most bio-available) and non-heme iron (from plant sources). Contrary to popular belief, although vegetarians and vegans don't eat any heme iron, they have been found to be no more likely to be deficient in iron. The body can make do with non-heme iron from plant sources, particularly if you have a high intake of vitamin C-rich fruit and vegetables as the vitamin C helps with iron absorption.

L-theanine

This is an amino acid found in green and black tea, which binds to brain cell receptors. Its calming effect has been found to reduce symptoms of anxiety and it is also associated with improved focus and concentration. In a 2012 study, those who took L-theanine performed better in a cognitive task than a placebo group.[44]

L-tryptophan

A plant-derived amino acid, L-tryptophan is the precursor to the 'happy hormone' serotonin. The brain needs it to make serotonin,[45] so too little has been found to be linked to mood disorders and sleep problems. Sleep quality has a huge impact on brain function, so anything you can do to support healthy sleep will benefit your brain. Dietary sources of L-tryptophan include dark-green leafy vegetables, salmon, bananas, nuts, seeds, oats, beans and lentils, tofu, red meat, turkey and eggs.

Magnesium L-threonate

The most absorbable of the magnesium supplements, because it crosses the blood–brain barrier, magnesium L-threonate has been proven to have a beneficial impact on brain function in a range of ways. It has been found to improve memory and cognitive function and improve sleep. In a 2013 Chinese study, supplementation with magnesium L-threonate was observed to help restore impaired memory damage.[46]

Omega-3 fatty acids

The brain is 60 per cent fat and your brain needs several types of long chain omega-3 fatty acids to function optimally: alpha-linolenic acid or ALA (not to be confused with the other ALA, alpha-lipoic acid produced by the body, see above) found in plant oils, plus eicosapentaenoic acid (EPA), docosahexaenoic acid (DHA) and docosapentaenoic acid (DPA), all commonly found in oily fish. A 2015 review of evidence into the impact of omega 3's on the brain found that different omega-3's worked in tandem to offset neurodegenerative symptoms.[47] The review concluded that preliminary evidence suggests the greatest benefit may been seen with DHA in non-cognitively impaired older people. Krill oil, made from the tiny crustaceans that feed on the phytoplankton in the depths of the oceans, is the purest source of omega-3. It has been extensively studied and found to reduce inflammation better than fish oils.

Phosphatidylserine (PS)

This fatty substance, which contains amino and fatty acids, is essential for efficient cell signalling in the brain. It is known that levels decline with age and some studies have found that dietary supplementation has been seen to improve memory. A 2014 review[48] of evidence drawn from 127 clinical trials concluded that exogenous PS, 300–800 mg daily, is absorbed efficiently in humans. It crosses the blood–brain barrier, and safely slows, halts, or reverses biochemical alterations and structural deterioration in nerve cells. It supports human cognitive functions, including the abilities to learn, focus and concentrate, reason and problem-solve, communicate, as well as acquire language. Phosphatidylserine is a common ingredient in combined nootropic supplements.

Resveratrol

This is one of a group of compounds called polyphenols that are thought to act like antioxidants. Found in red grapes and red wine, resveratrol can help to stop memory loss. A study in rats at A&M University, Texas, USA, showed that it decreased inflammation in the hippocampus, the area of the brain related to memory, and boosted the numbers of neurons.

Vincamine/Vinpocetine

Vincamine is a supplement obtained from the leaves of the *vinca minor* (periwinkle). Vinpocetine is a synthetic form that has a similar structure. Evidence for its brain-specific benefits is mixed, although some research suggests that supplementation can increase brain blood flow (which boosts oxygen delivery) and memory. A 2007 Hungarian study into the benefits of vinpocetine[49] found that supplementation significantly improved cerebral blood flow, and showed improvements in patients' cognitive function, demonstrated by performance in psychometric tests.

Vitamins

B Vitamins There are eight different B vitamins, and many play a crucial role in brain health, particularly in mental energy and brain-repair processes. All are important but most research has concentrated on three: B6, B12 and B9 (folate, the natural form, or folic acid, its synthetic form). For an overview of their wide-ranging benefits, a 2016 review of clinical data is worth reading.[50]

Vitamin B12 is particularly important for brain health and is one that most of us need to consider taking as a daily supplement. Unlike some vitamins, B12 is stored by the body for long-term use, which means that deficiency can take time to develop. Vegans are particularly at risk of deficiency, as B12 is only found in animal products. Anyone who consumes little or no animal products should take it as a supplement, although the amount found in a multivitamin should be sufficient as the required daily amount is small. The symptoms of B12 deficiency can include memory deficiency and low mood and dementia. Vitamin B12 increases the levels of GABA neurotransmitters in the brain; low GABA levels are associated with a variety of neurological disorders.

Vitamin C Neurodegenerative diseases, such as dementia, are characterised by high levels of oxidative stress in the brain, so antioxidants such as vitamin C, or ascorbic acid, can help to counteract this. Vitamin C also supports healthy brain function, as it plays a part in several enzyme reactions, it helps the body to absorb key nutrients, including iron, and boosts production of neurotransmitters.[51]

Vitamin E Another important antioxidant, vitamin E is widely fêted as an anti-ageing wonder. It has been found to play a role in offsetting age-related degeneration and oxidative damage in the brain, and elsewhere in the body, although research reveals a somewhat inconclusive picture.[52] However, in a 1999 American study[53] that looked at 445 multi-ethnic older people, low levels of vitamin E were found to correlate with poor memory recall. Importantly, make sure you supplement with natural vitamin E – not the synthetic forms (all-rac-alpha-tocopherol-acetate or dl-alpha-tocopherol) as there are serious questions about safety.

Vitamin D The main source of this vitamin is sunlight, and in the northern hemisphere the angle of the sun can be too low for UVB rays to penetrate your skin and trigger production. So, unsurprisingly, some 75 per cent of the UK's population is believed to be deficient in vitamin D.[54] Some foods, such as oily fish, contain vitamin D, but it is a good idea to supplement through the winter to ensure your stores don't run too low. Low levels can wreak havoc in the brain (and the rest of the body). Every tissue and cell (including those that make up your brain tissue) has a vitamin D receptor, and deficiency is linked with everything from depression to autoimmune diseases such as multiple sclerosis and diabetes.[55] Recently, vitamin D's biologically active form has been found to have neuroprotective effects, including assisting in the clearance of amyloid plaques (the build-up of which is a sign of Alzheimer's disease).[56]

Zinc

A mineral most widely known for its immune-boosting benefits and the role it plays in the production of healthy sex hormones, zinc is also key to a range of functions in the brain,[57] particularly synaptic and axonal activity. In pregnant and lactating mothers, healthy levels of zinc have been found to play an important role in supporting the brain function of the foetus and infant. Zinc deficiency in children is associated with a range of impaired neurological symptoms. Dietary sources include meat, seeds, nuts, legumes and dairy products.

ASEA Redox supplement

Oxidative stress is one of the causes of the death of brain nerve cells. If neurons in specific areas of the brain are not replaced as they die off, then that area will begin to malfunction. By increasing redox signalling (the transduction of signal coding for cellular processes, which keeps oxidative stress to a minimum), you can reduce inflammation in the brain and restore brain cells to health. The number of redox signalling molecules decreases with age – they can reduce by 90 per cent by the time you reach the age of 70. ASEA Redox is a proprietary supplement that is said to contain active redox signalling molecules, which can cross the blood–brain barrier and enable neurons to repair themselves.

Did you know – about Neuroplasticity support supplements?

Researched Nutritionals makes a supplement – BDNF Essentials – designed to help your brain activity as you age. Only available through a medical practitioner, it contains specific herbs, mushroom and nutrients found to have protective properties that help memory, concentration and cognitive processing. www.researchednutritionals.com

Exercise: How to move

Exercise delivers increased oxygen and energy to your brain, and has been identified as a key way to encourage neuroplasticity – the formation of new neurons and the strengthening and growth of neural pathways in the brain. It can expand the size of the hippocampus, the area of the brain associated with memory. Research published in Proceedings of the National Academy of Sciences of the United States showed that cardio and weight training increased the volume of the hippocampus by two per cent and reversed age-related volume shrinkage by one to two years.

Exercise is recognised to have a preventative influence in older adults at risk of developing dementia. The UK's Alzheimer's Society looked at the results of 11 studies, and found that regular exercise reduced the risk of developing dementia by 30 per cent.[58] Other studies show that regular exercise boosts higher-level brain function, and reduces a range of aspects of cognitive decline. Another study by researchers at the Radiological Society of North America took a group of older adults suffering mild cognitive impairment and split them into two groups.[59] For a six-month period, half the group was directed to stretch regularly and the other to exercise four times a week. At the end of the study, fMRI (functional magnetic resonance imaging) showed that the exercise group showed increased brain volume and grey matter in their brains and showed improved executive function, an important measure of overall brain function.

Why does exercise have such a dramatic impact?

In part, it is the effect of exercise on a protein called brain derived neurotrophic factor (BDNF), a substance that encourages brain cell repair and resilience, increasing the capacity of the mitochondria – the energy power plants of your cells. Exercise encourages the production of BDNF, ensuring the brain has a healthy supply of new neurons.[60] In other words, exercise helps your brain repair itself – which also explains why brain scans of older people who exercise show less age-related deterioration in the brain.[61]

Regular cardiovascular exercise that elevates your heart rate has been demonstrated, in multiple studies, to be one of the best ways to encourage neuroplasticity in the brain. Even 30 minutes a day of moderate exercise has been found to increase the production of new synapses.[62]

The greatest benefit appears to result from interval, or varied pace, training, during which you alternate fast-paced, maximum-effort intervals of exercise with slower recovery periods. But most effective of all is high intensity interval training, or 'HIIT'.[63] After interval training, and especially following an HIIT session, levels of BDNF in the brain rise dramatically. In a study at the Mayo clinic, USA, a group of over 65s who started an HIIT regime saw a reduction in age-related deterioration of muscle cells. Research published in *Cell Metabolism* found a substantial mitochondrial boost following a three-month HIIT programme. Mitochondrial capacity was increased by 49 per cent in younger participants, and by 69 per cent in older people – aerobic exercise reversed the ageing of the mitochondria.[64]

Cognitive decline is the result of withering of connections and the death of neurons. So, anything that increases BDNF, mitochondrial capacity and neuroplasticity is an effective antidote. In the past, neurogenesis, the forming of new brain cells, was believed to be all but impossible in adults, but research now shows that neurogenesis does occur in adult brains in the areas of the brain responsible for governing memory and learning. Why such bursts of effort and exertion seem to have the biggest positive impact on BDNF levels is still under investigation,[65] but it has been suggested that the shorter the time you spend exercising, the less the impact of oxidative stress.

As well as delivering twice the improvement in BDNF, HIIT training has been found to be a better way to combat central obesity. This is good news for the brain, as a higher waist-to-hip ratio has been found to be linked to brain shrinkage and a decrease in grey matter, the part of the brain containing most of your nerve cells and involved in memory, hearing, seeing, speech and decision making.[66]

Combinations that provide the greatest brain benefit

Alternate regular HIIT sessions (or stop-start activity) with slower-paced walking. The HIIT programme will increase blood flow and oxygen levels to the brain, while a walk is the perfect time to try a moving meditation, or you can use it to catch up on some quality conversation with a friend, or bond with your dog. All of these activities have been proven to reduce anxiety and boost mood, too, so you'll get double the brain benefit. Do them somewhere green and the benefit is even greater (see page 169).

Opt for four cardio sessions where you try fast–slow training, per week – 20 to 30 minutes per session is enough to feel the benefit. Combine this with two sessions of breathing-based yoga, and you'll be covering all the bases. Vigorous exercise stimulates the release of anandamide, and the sense of euphoric wellbeing that comes with a healthy workout – what jogging enthusiasts refer to as a 'runner's high' – is due to elevated levels of this natural brain endocannabinoid. The endocannabinoid system in the brain is also believed to help mediate emotions, consolidate memory and coordinate movement.

Apart from the direct effects that exercise has on cognition, its indirect effects – improved sleep quality, reduced hypertension and stress and improved mental health – are an added bonus.

Build your own mini HIIT circuit

You can build your own circuit around any cardiovascular activity – brisk walking, cycling, rowing, running – and do it at home or in a gym.

- Choose your activity

- Warm up with 5 minutes of light exertion – stand tall and circle your arms backwards, one after the other for 30 seconds.

- Do 20 seconds of your chosen activity at a high intensity – really go for it.

- Rest for 10 seconds

- Repeat 20 seconds of your high-intensity exercise, alternating with the 10-second rest period, four more times.

- Do some cool-down stretches.

Now you're done.

Strength training

Most research on the connection between exercise and brain health has focused on aerobic exercise, but as we age, particularly in our 70s and 80s, the potential risk of injury or a fall could outweigh the benefits. Improvement in strength, balance, coordination and reaction speeds also boost the brain, and a 2010 study revealed that older adults who participated in a once-weekly strength-training exercise programme showed sustained cognitive benefits as long as one year after the training.[67]

Cross crawl programme

Cross crawl is a form of exercise in which you use opposite sides of the body – right arm to left leg, and then left arm to right leg, across the midline of your body – to boost physical coordination and brain function. This type of exercise not only builds core strength and stabilises balance, but it also releases stress, boosts energy levels and clarity of thought, and helps with focus and spatial and touch awareness.

The movements stimulate the integration and development of your brain and nervous system and fire up neural pathways in the right and left side of your brain at the same time. Cross crawl also builds a connective path between both sides of the brain, smoothing the way for electrical impulses and information to move between the two. Ten minutes of cross crawl exercises each day strengthens communication between body and brain.

How to do cross crawl

● **1** Stand with your feet apart and your arms outstretched and parallel to the ground.

● **2** Move your weight onto your right foot, lift your left knee and touch it with your right hand. Put your left foot down and recentre your weight.

● **3** Immediately shift your weight over to your left foot; lift your right knee and touch it with your left hand.

● **4** Repeat 10 times, then relax.

Green therapy

If you can find an open green space to do your workout, so much the better. A report from researchers at the University of East Anglia, UK, using data relating to 290 million people, found that living close to green space, and spending time in it, correlates with a significant reduction in levels of cortisol (the stress hormone).[68] Researchers at New Mexico Highlands University, USA, also found that, after walking outside, blood flow to the brain increased. They found the effect related to 'foot impact', not just the increased oxygen and cardiovascular exertion, as walking was found to boost blood flow to the brain more than cycling. In the study, running, which has a stronger foot strike, came out top.

Regular long walks build greater grey matter volume in your brain, which is also associated with a reduced risk of cognitive impairment.[69] So, walk as much as you can and ideally in green spaces.

Wake-up yoga

Even 10 minutes of yoga first thing in the morning will make a huge difference to your wellbeing. A 2015 study used fMRI to look at the brains of older yogis and non-yogis and found physical differences in the brains of the yogis that were 'neuroprotective'. The results were most pronounced in those who did a combination of yoga and meditation, and the more time they spent doing yoga, the greater the benefit.[70] Research from UCLA showed that a three month course of yoga and meditation was more effective than memory games or crosswords at reducing the cognitive difficulties of patients with Alzheimer's disease. You might think you don't have time to get to a class, but there are so many great YouTube videos now you can do it at home. Even a few simple sun salutations will not only boost fitness,[71] but mood and memory, too.[72]

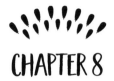

CHAPTER 8

THE GUT-BRAIN, HEART-BRAIN, AND HORMONES

'As your trillions of new connections continually form and re-form, the distinctive pattern means that no one like you has ever existed, or will ever exist again. The experience of your conscious awareness, right now, is unique to you... We're not fixed. From cradle to grave, we are works in progress.'

DAVID EAGLEMAN AUTHOR AND NEUROSCIENTIST

Despite the recent explosion of research into the relationship between our brain and various other systems within the body (vascular, digestive, and so on) the average person's understanding of how these key organs interconnect is still sketchy at best. When most people think about the brain, they see it in isolation and picture it floating inside their skull. Anyone who studied basic human biology at school will know that the brain connects to the body via the brainstem, which sits at the top of the spinal cord, and it's the brain stem that controls the flow of information from the body in and out of the brain (see also Chapter 1). The general perception is that the brain and the body are somehow separate, linked, but independent entities, and this view needs to shift if you are to reboot your brain effectively.

The advent of functional magnetic resonance imaging (fMRI) means that researchers can actually observe the brain–body connectivity in all its complexity. They can trace the intricate web of neural pathways throughout the body, and observe areas outside the brain, such as the gut and the heart, where dense collections of neurons also reside. These satellite clusters of neurons are now the subject of intense interest and study.

Brain scans can show what the activities of the body, from a strenuous bike ride to watching TV or keeping hydrated *do* to your brain. Everything from your activities to the noises you are exposed to on a daily basis, or the types of fillings in your teeth, can have a profound impact on brain function.

We need to think outside the box

There is plenty you can do to influence your brain for the better. Up to now, we thought that cerebral activities – from jigsaws, crossword puzzles, and mental arithmetic to political thinking – were the best ways to 'exercise' or improve the brain. Whilst you can benefit from these activities, everything we are learning about neuroscience now points to a far more holistic reality.

The word 'brain' more accurately describes an organ with 'outposts' (from the gut to the heart and the spine) that also has a two-way relationship with your hormones, or chemical messengers. The health of each and every aspect of your body plays a part in the balance and wellbeing of your brain, and your sensory organs – eyes, ears, nose, skin and mouth – are primary sources of data.

Once you accept that the brain exists within your body, and is influenced by, and influences, every part of it all the time, you start to see that the relationship between the brain and the rest of your body is entirely symbiotic.

The gut-brain

It is the connection between the gut and the brain – or the gut-brain – that I am asked about most often. Whenever I post about it on my blog, Reboothealth (www.reboothealth.co.uk), I get a higher than average number of questions, and readers repeatedly tell me they want to know more.

Perhaps, fittingly, it makes intuitive sense to us. Many of us 'sense' things through our 'gut' before any information is filtered by our brain. You will know the phrase 'gut feeling', an experiential signpost of a two-way channel of communication between our brain and gut. Newspaper headlines about the growing body of gut-brain research have focused on the mounting evidence that our microbiome (gut flora) influences everything from depression to the risk of dementia – proving we are what we eat, in a mental as well as a physical sense. But because gut flora is so complex, it is likely to be some time before its impact on our bodies as a whole, and on our brains, is fully understood.

What is the gut flora, or microbiome?

A staggering 100 trillion microorganisms live in the human gut, and they are estimated to weigh up to 1kg (2$^1/_4$lb) – that's a bag of potatoes.[1] These microorganisms are also thought to contain 150 times more genes than the human genome, so there is much we don't know about them. However, we do know that gut bacteria have a profound impact on our immune system – the immune tissues in the digestive tract are the largest and most complex part of the immune system – and that there are millions of neurons embedded in the gut walls. These neurons, or gut 'brain' cells, are not only there to signal the more obvious functions of digestion like satiation or sickness, they also help you think and remember. Think about where you feel feelings of dread, or anticipation – it's in the pit of your stomach. This isn't an imagined displacement of the brain's feelings into another part of the body, you really are feeling emotions there.

Your brain health is determined from early childhood, partly inherited from your genetic makeup. It's the same with your gut. Scientists are beginning to understand that not only the food you eat, but also the microbes in your stomach and intestines – some of which are also inherited – affect your mental health too. They can direct the way you think and behave as well as indicate the likelihood of your developing certain mental illnesses. Anxiety, depression, ADHD and memory problems have been shown to be linked to problems with the gut flora.

It may soon be possible to identify mental health and brain diseases by analysing the microbes in your gut, and perhaps, by altering the balance of those microbes and introducing specifically targeted new species, rebalance and even cure those diseases. There's not much you can do to alter and change your genes, but when this new research becomes medical fact, the fate of your mind could well be in your own hands. With specially designed brain biotics you can literally change the chemical balance of your mind. This is the cutting edge of brain medicine.

What are brain biotics?

These are, essentially, probiotics with brain-changing properties. The term 'psychobiotic' was coined in 2013 by Ted Dinan from the University of Cork, Ireland. It was originally used to describe specific live microbes that, when eaten in enough quantity, can alter the composition of the bacteria in your gut to positively affect your mental health.

The understanding of the word psychobiotic has been extended to include any probiotic and prebiotic that affects brain function and behaviour via changes made to the gut microbiome – a number of these have been shown to make significant differences to mood and mental activity.

We know that there is a connection between anxiety, depression and other psychiatric and neurodegenerative illnesses and the state of our gut health. Boost the numbers of these bacterial brain, or 'psycho', biotics, and you reduce the proportion of the 'bad' bacteria that create the problems – improving your mental and digestive health at the same time. But, bear in mind that not all psychobiotics are beneficial. For example, antibiotics, antipsychotics and antidepressants have been shown to permanently change the terrain of the gut, causing neurochemical and behavioural changes that affect the brain – and not necessarily in a good way.

The discovery of these psychobiotics means that, to a certain degree, the health of our brain is back in our own control.[2] For a breakdown of which psychobiotic does what, check the chart on pages 267–69 in the references section.

Tailored treatments and faecal transplants

Specialist centres and some supplement companies are ahead of the curve in the fast-developing world of probiotic technology. Research shows that individually customised bacterial 'prescriptions' are far more effective at reducing symptoms of digestive disorders than conventional medical treatments and 'off the shelf' probiotics.

For the brave, cutting-edge treatments such as faecal transplants, in which a patient receives faecal bacteria from a healthy donor, have been remarkably successful in treating chronic conditions such as Crohn's disease and colitis, and bacterial infections, such as c. difficile. It may sound disgusting, but a faecal transplant is a last resort for many.[3]

I recently met with the husband and wife team who run the Taymount Clinic, a pioneering faecal transplant clinic in Hertfordshire, UK. Although most of their work is with patients suffering from chronic digestive disorders, such as colitis, Crohn's and IBS, there have been promising results in improving cognitive function for a range of patients too. [4] Studies are underway to assess the potential for the treatment of degenerative brain diseases, including Alzheimer's and Parkinson's diseases, with faecal transplants.

Neurotransmitters – the brain's messenger chemicals

These are the chemical transmitters released by nerve cells, which not only carry messages from one cell to another, but also stimulate nearby glands or muscles (see also reference section). Your gut has its own 'second brain', your enteric nervous system, and the microbes in your gut produce more than 30 neurotransmitters, including serotonin, dopamine, acetylcholine and gamma-aminobutyric acid (GABA), so if you want to actively and positively affect your brain function, choose your bacteria carefully.[5]

Your neurons, the nerve cells in your brain, are stimulated and boosted by neurotransmitters in different ways and more than 90 per cent of your serotonin, your 'happy' hormone, and 50 per cent of your dopamine is made by the gut bacteria. It is thought that the neurotransmitters trigger cells in the gut wall lining to produce molecules that send messages to the brain. They also boost BDNF (brain derived neurotrophic factor), which is the protein that calms the brain and creates new brain cells, or at least it does in mice![6]

More information about the effects of different neurotransmitters can be found on pages 254–265 of the reference section.

Bacteria that make brain chemicals[7]

Bacteria	Neural messengers
Bacillus	Dopamine, noradrenaline (norepinephrine)
Bifidobacterium	Gamma-aminobutyric acid (GABA)
Enterococcus	Serotonin
Escherichia	Noradrenaline (norepinephrine), serotonin
Lactobacillus	Acetylcholine, Gamma-aminobutyric acid (GABA)
Streptococcus	Serotonin

The bacteria-serotonin link

Most of the body's serotonin, the neurotransmitter responsible for mood, is produced in the gut, and we also know that treatment with probiotics has been found to significantly reduce symptoms of depression. A 2018 study by a team from Tehran University Medical School, Iran, concluded that there is now a great body of evidence indicating that pathophysiological pathways involved in the pathogenesis of depression are influenced by disturbance in the equilibrium of the gut microbiota. For the purposes of the trial, 110 depressive patients were separated into three groups.[8] At the outset, all of them were tested using Beck Depression Scores – a commonly used diagnostic tool for depression. For a period of eight weeks, one group was given a combination of two live-culture probiotics (at a strength of 10 billion CFUs), the second group had a prebiotic supplement (galactooligosaccharide), and those in the third group were given a placebo. During the process, serum L-tryptophan, branch chain amino acid and kynurenine levels were all measured. Kynurenine is a 'catabolic' metabolite that plays an important role in the gut-brain axis, as the body needs it to be able to break down L-tryptophan, a key amino acid required in serotonin production.

The 81 patients who completed the trial (28 in the probiotic group, 27 in the prebiotic group, and 26 of the placebos) retook the Beck Depression test after treatment. Those in the probiotic group saw a significant improvement in depressive symptoms, but there was no significant improvement for patients in either of the other groups. The probiotic group also saw a significant decrease in their kynurenine/L-tryptophan ratio, an indicator that the neurochemistry underlying their depressive symptoms was improved as a result of the changes in microbiota (suggesting that their biological 'need' for L-tryptophan was lessened).

Action plan

- **Choose a good probiotic supplement** Make sure that it is one that will help your specific symptoms. There are plenty of mass-produced synthesised products, but there are smaller companies who can offer combinations of naturally produced probiotic strains, such as Micromax, which has more than 60 strains (healthy.co.uk). Consult my list of probiotics and their specific brain benefits to choose the right ones for you (see pages 266–69).

- **Look for Bravo GcMAF yogurt** This is a probiotic yoghurt that contains 42 essential probiotics and GcMAF, one of the most powerful of the immune system activators. GcMAF stimulates production of macrophages, immune cells that attack and destroy bacteria, viruses, fungi and parasites, boosts immunity and prevents metastasis of cancer cells. www.bravoprobiotic.co.uk

- **Take a natural anti-inflammatory** Try aloe vera, curcumin or evening primrose oil.

- **Cut sugar out of your diet** Sugar triggers the release of inflammatory cytokines that impair cognitive clarity.[9]

- **Exercise more** This will boost your mitochondria (see page 30).

- **Consider a ketogenic diet** This very low-carb, high-fat diet cuts inflammation in the brain, reducing stress.[10]

The heart-brain

Another exciting area of research is the connection between the heart and brain, which has resulted in the emergence of a hybrid field of neurocardiology.[11] A number of studies have researched the correlation between vascular diseases and cognitive decline that leads to dementia. Studies have also looked at the role of the brain–heart connection and its impact on healthy emotional attachment following trauma and grief. Romantic notions such as dying of a 'broken heart,' or anecdotal reports of people who become 'cut off' from emotion, unable to feel love, sadness, or desire after a traumatic experience, appear to make sense physiologically, too.

The heart has its own complex nervous system. It has a network of 40,000 neurons and neurotransmitters that operate in a similar way to those in the brain. This so-called 'heart-brain' – not a scientific term, but nevertheless a useful one – can feel, understand, learn and remember and is intuitive. Think of it as an information-processing system that communicates with the brain in your skull via the central nervous system. Human beings are essentially energy systems, and emotions are the keys to 'reading' that energy.

When your heart rhythm is regular, relaxed and functioning well, research shows it sends a signal throughout the body, including the brain, which promotes wellbeing and improves mental clarity and intuitive decision making.[12] We also know that when a person feels an emotion deeply, it is experienced in their heart, which then reports back to the brain. In contrast, an irregular heart rhythm is linked to the onset of dementia.[13]

The Heart Math Institute, California, USA has been looking at the effects on the brain of coherent heartbeats for more than

20 years. When your heart rate variability (HRV) is regular and coherent, it brings your brain into line too. There is an energetic, electric connection between them. Humans are electric beings and emotions are frequencies that give us feedback to what is happening around us – both 'out there' and 'in here'. The brain's alpha and beta waves synchronise with the heart's rhythm and appear to be directed by intention.

How you can help

Brain coherence leads to balance of the neurotransmitters dopamine and serotonin. Meditation is a way of accessing that brain coherence, but it should always be done first thing in the morning, as close to waking up as you can, when you have just recently emerged from the alpha state. The coherent human heart and the slowest of the frequencies of the earth's magnetic field are the same frequency – 0.1Hz.[14] (See Chapter 9 for more on meditation.)

If you stop leading your life principally through thoughts, and begin to read your environment through emotions and feelings instead, your world, and your brain, will change. Emotions regulate your brain, enabling it to make decisions based on these frequencies long before your conscious mind receives them. Look again at Chapter 6 for advice on regulating your brain.

Hormones and the brain

Finally, there is much to explore in the impact of hormones, your chemical messengers, on your brain, and vice versa. The brain – through the pituitary gland, or 'master' gland of the hormone, or endocrine, system that sits beneath it – controls and communicates with your thyroid gland, adrenal glands, testes and ovaries. As a result, reproduction and sexual function, metabolism, weight gain and stress response all depend on healthy brain function.

Hormones, and the glands that secrete and respond to them, are in constant communication with one another. Some hormones (such as endorphins that relieve pain, and growth hormone that supports the growth and regeneration of healthy bones and muscles) are produced in the brain by the hypothalamus, which sits next to the pituitary gland. Others rely on signals from the pituitary gland to tell other hormonal glands in the body how much to produce and when.

Healthy hormonal balance is also impacted by inflammatory processes in the body and brain. Excessive stress or chronic illness can trigger inflammation, which disrupts the production and release of cortisol and other stress-related hormones. This in turn may trigger memory problems and mood disorders, and contribute to high levels of anxiety and depression. When your immune system is activated, and your inflammatory markers are high, hormonal production and regulation are compromised. This process is complicated by the feelings associated with hormones and the way the feelings mediate our experience of the world around us.

We know that feelings (happiness, elation, sadness, arousal, anger) and energy levels operate in a symbiotic feedback loop with the endocrine system and the brain directs it.

But hormones dictate brain function and mood to a greater extent than we give them credit for. The main memory hormone is pregnenolone, which makes oestrogen, dehydroepiandrosterone (DHEA) and cortisol; oestrogen is 'memory for women', testosterone in particular is 'memory for men'. If your pregnenolone levels are low and you take action to boost them, expect your mental acuity to sharpen. Simply understanding the complexity of the relationship is an important first step. Hormone production has been shown to be responsive to physical and environmental change, for example, we produce more testosterone when we exercise, but also when we argue – further evidence that targeted action can actively benefit our brains.

Action plan

- **Get your hormone levels checked** Consult a specialist and ask them to check your hormones; some do this with a blood test, others check urine or saliva. Testing timetables will vary too.

- **Consider supplements** You can supplement with bio-identical hormones if your levels are low.

- **Reduce your stress levels** Pay attention to your stress levels, and take steps to reduce them if necessary, as raised stress levels can throw your hormones off balance, and trigger brain fog, memory problems, anxiety and depression.

- **Take omega-3 fatty acid supplements** Research indicates that omega-3s control cortisol and epinephrine, so taking supplements can reduce mental stress.[15]

- **Sort your sleep** Your brain needs 7–7 $1/2$ hours of good-quality, uninterrupted sleep for optimal hormone balance. Poor quality and quantity of sleep has been linked to imbalances of the hypothalamus and pituitary gland.[16] (See Chapter 9 for help on how to improve sleep.)

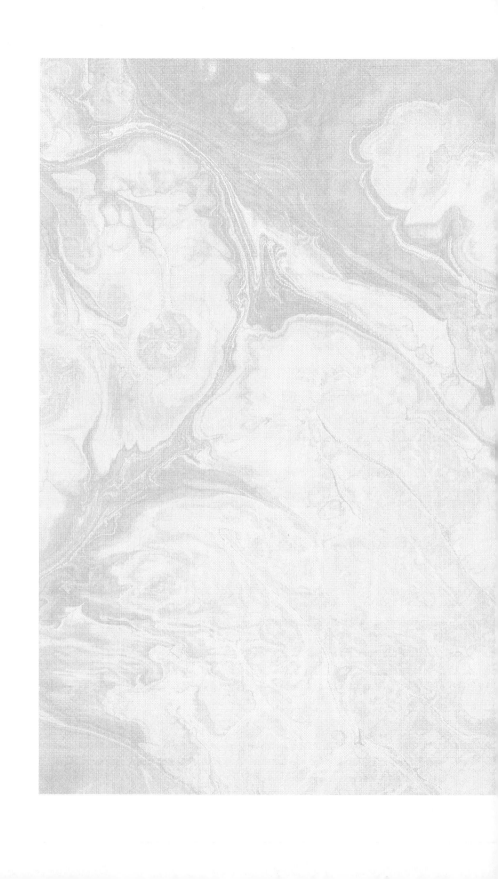

STEP THREE

—

BOOST *your* Brain

'Transformation is always an inside out process.'

HEIDI DUPREE, AUTHOR AND ENERGY HEALER

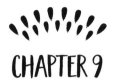

CHAPTER 9

DAILY PRACTICES

*'Your brain loves habits because they are simple,
structured, well-known, energy efficient and automatic.'*

STAN JACOBS, AUTHOR

I n the introduction, I touched on the ways that our environment
shapes our brain and the impact of our lifestyle, behaviours and
habits on mental wellbeing and brain function. The emerging
science of epigenetics – the study of changes in organisms
caused by modification of gene expression rather than alteration
of the genetic code – goes some way to explain how key genes
express themselves, or are switched 'off' or 'on', in response not
only to the environmental signals, but also to what you think and
feel. The brain uses its own activity as data for the continuous
process of making sense of what is happening to us. And through
its plasticity (its capacity to go on changing and create new
pathways even though in general it prefers to stay the same),
new thoughts, behaviours and environmental stimuli will change
its structure, as they each become part of its database.

Time to create new directions

Once you have reduced the stress-load on your brain by implementing the suggestions in the first section of this book (Chapters 3 to 6), you'll have the resources to set about creating new, positive habits and daily practices that will prime your brain through its neuroplasticity. It's time to create what you positively want – the adaptive way of getting rid of what you don't want. Evidence is beginning to suggest that by making these changes you can reduce your rate of cognitive decline and encourage the formation of healthy new pathways. As these habits become embedded you can feel the way they improve your mood. A virtuous circle takes the place of the earlier vicious circle and this cascades through all your bodily functions – you feel better.

Think of this as 'brain hygiene'. You already understand the necessity of twice daily brushing and flossing and avoiding too many sugary snacks to keep tooth decay at bay, or hand-washing to reduce the risk of bacterial and viral contamination. Look at the importance of sticking to positive lifestyle habits, such as daily mindfulness meditation, exercise, active gratitude, spending time outdoors, and a regular, healthy sleep, as similarly essential to maintaining your brain in optimal condition.

When you're pushed for time and struggling to keep up with the day-to-day demands, the idea of making space for a load of new healthy habits can feel onerous. I've distilled the research and recommendations for you and transformed it into minimum-effort, maximum-benefit practices. They are designed to fit around your life and take up as little time as possible. Declutter your brain, release yesterday's stresses, and your today will flow more smoothly. Science proves it.

Mindfulness meditation

*'Meditation is not just blissing out under a mango tree.
It completely changes your brain and therefore changes
what you are.'*

MATTHIEU RICARD, BUDDHIST MONK

Unless you've been living in a cave for the past ten years, you'll have seen the headlines about the many brain benefits of mindfulness meditation and you may well have tried one of the mindfulness apps. It has long been understood that people who practice mindfulness meditation regularly report feeling calmer and happier as a result, and take fewer sick days than colleagues who don't.[1] In the US military, it has been found that even the toughest soldiers respond more effectively under the stresses of simulated battle conditions if they have incorporated mindfulness practices into their daily routines.

Before the advent of fMRI (functional magnetic resonance imaging), those studying the impact of meditation relied mainly on self-reported measures of mental wellbeing and performance and/or they measured the impact with cognitive tests that asked people to respond to a series of standardised questions. But fMRI has enabled researchers to observe what is going on inside the brain during meditation, and they have seen how new brain cells grow (neurogenesis) in the brains of regular meditators over time, and can document physical changes in key brain regions. The changes are really quite remarkable. American neuroscientist and author, Dr Andrew Newberg, has led a number of pioneering studies that focus on the impact of various religious and spiritual practices on the brain. In his paper using data based on brain images of Tibetan monks during meditation, he reports that their frontal lobes lit up (the area of the brain responsible for both problem solving and impulse control, amongst other things), whilst simultaneously, the parietal lobes showed a drop in activity. Reduced activity in the parietal lobe has been proven to correlate with a loss of a sense of self, a feeling of 'oneness' that Newberg says: 'results in the blurring of the boundary between self and others'.

This explains why meditation has been found to make a person more empathetic, better attuned to the feelings of others and better able to regulate their own moods and thoughts. Meditators have also been shown to have higher volumes of brain tissue, reduced brain inflammation, well-balanced neurotransmitters and less stress.[2]

Brain scans have also shown that the brain regions related to attention and sensory processing are more developed[3] in people who meditate regularly, so they are more attuned to the here and now. A greater capacity for 'noticing' has been linked with higher cognitive performance, as 'noticing' is the domain of our working memory. We rely on this ability to help retain information.

Meditation is highly recommended if you are one of the one in four people who suffers from mental ill health, including anxiety or depression. In a 2013 study, 93 people who had been diagnosed with generalised anxiety disorder were assigned to a mindfulness group for eight weeks, whilst another group received stress management advice.[4] Those who did the mindfulness programme experienced a significantly greater reduction in their symptoms. Similarly, research from the University of Oxford found that a mindfulness intervention was more effective at helping prevent a recurrence of depressive episodes than antidepressant medication.[5]

How to meditate

'Do or do not. There is no try.'

YODA, LEGENDARY JEDI MASTER

Whether this is your first time meditating, or you've explored it before, the key thing to remember is that while the benefits are instant, they are also incremental. Committing to regular meditation will deliver brain-changing benefits over time with practice (and patience). Don't expect it to be easy. It's quite normal to find that as soon as you try to still your mind, your brain is overrun by a whole load of unwanted and unwelcome thoughts. This is NOT a sign that you are 'bad' at meditation, or that it won't work for you. The key is to simply notice your distracting thoughts and move on, trying as far as you can to resist letting them lead you away from your breath, or your point of focus.

Morning meditation

This is a mindfulness meditation designed to energise you and help you improve your ability to focus and concentrate. It is a great way to counteract an anxious, over-busy brain. Aim to practise this for ten minutes as soon as possible after waking. You can meditate by listening to breathing or sound.

➥ Using breathing

1 Sit with a relaxed, upright spine and close your eyes.

2 Begin to focus on your breath, draw the air deep down to the very bottom of your lungs. Notice the sensation of air flowing into your nostrils for a count of four, pause for a moment at the top of the breath.

3 Exhale for a count of four. Repeat.

4 Repeat the in and out breaths as above for 10 minutes, focusing on them at all times. Whenever thoughts intrude, draw your attention back to your breath.

➤ Using sound

Sit with your eyes closed and breathe in and out as above. Don't worry too much about counting as you breathe, instead focus your attention fully on your hearing. Pay attention to the sounds going on around you, noticing them as they occur. Concentrate for a while on the ones closest to you, then extend your hearing out into the wider world. Note each one mentally, and keep listening for the next sound.

Wind-down meditation

This is a loving-kindness meditation, designed to improve your self-compassion. Research shows that those who practice this type of meditation report decreased rumination (the type of negative thought associated with depression and anxiety), and increased self-esteem. Even more fascinatingly, there is research to show that the benefits of this meditation include improved physical wellbeing. In a 2005 study, a randomised group of people suffering from back pain who practised loving-kindness meditation daily, saw greater reductions in their pain than those who received standard treatment.[6]

➤ What to do

1 Sit quietly somewhere and close your eyes. Bring to your mind a quality within you that you are proud of, or feel good about.

2 Breathe steadily and focus on the quality. Picture yourself in your mind's eye.

3 Identify some positive statement(s) you would like to focus on: they should demonstrate self-compassion and should take the form of wishes for yourself that begin with the phrase: 'May I be...' Then, for example, ...happy ...healthy ...safe ...loved'. In your mind, or aloud if you want to, recite the phrase, or phrases that resonate most with you. Focus on opening your heart and sending yourself the emotion, or quality, you are focusing on. Once you can feel the positive energy and can fill yourself with self-compassion, you can move onto somebody else.

4 Next, call somebody to mind who you like, and who could do with some compassion, and send them some loving-kindness. And follow the same process.

5 Finally, do the same with a difficult person in your life, and follow the same process.

Laughter

Spend more time with people that make you laugh. Laughter releases endorphins and opioid peptides in your brain calming and improving mood and reducing feelings of isolation.[7]

Learn something new

'When you stop learning, your brain starts dying.'

DR DANIEL AMEN

Use it or lose it; keep on learning. However old you are, your brain keeps changing, and the more you feed it new information, the sharper it will remain. Sign up for a painting class, a lecture series or learn a new language. Physical activities that involve an additional challenge requiring total concentration, such as martial arts where quick reactions are essential, or dance routines where responding to your partner and focus on new routines are key, all boost brain health.

Brain HQ (www.brainhq.com) is an app with brain exercises backed by more than 100 scientific studies that have been shown to help with growing and stimulating neural pathways. Doing these exercises shows a reversal of age-related neural slowing, a doubling, on average, in visual processing speed; and a 135 per cent increase in auditory processing speed.[8] There is also an average improvement of 10 years in memory and increased activity in areas of the brain associated with it, plus higher scores on measure of balance and gait.[9] So, think faster, focus better and remember more...

Use your non-dominant hand

Instead of the hand you are comfortable with, you can help your brain to integrate its two hemispheres and develop new neural pathways and connections by doing things with your other hand instead. Most of us are right-handed, some are left-handed, and a tiny minority can use both with equal ease. Your right hand is linked to the left hemisphere of your brain which controls the right side of your body and vice versa.

Studies using brain scans show that when you use your dominant hand, only one side of your brain is engaged. However, when you use the non-dominant hand, both hemispheres light up. Switch hands and you switch on your brain's unused pathways. Musicians often need to use both hands when they play. They engage both sides of their brain simultaneously, and as a result their corpus callosum is nine per cent larger.

Try switching over and using the non-dominant hand – do something different each day. Start with something easy. For example, brush your teeth with the opposite hand, or use a different hand to control your computer mouse.

Gratitude journalling

This daily practice fuses two proven brain-boosting practices, journalling and active gratitude, into one daily habit. The idea is simply that you spend ten minutes at the end of each day noting down three things that happened, or occurred to you during that day, that you feel grateful for. These can be as big or as small as you like and could relate to something that happened, or simply to a passing thought. Examples could include:

- Laughing with your child or grandchild

- Feeling the warmth on your back as you walked to the station, which reminded you spring was on its way

- Listening to a piece of music you love

- Good news about a project

Retraining your brain to notice the good things in your day-to-day life, big or small, will help you to become more optimistic, and the journalling itself has well-documented therapeutic benefits.[10]

Gratitude, however, is something that must be consciously cultivated by regular practice.[11] Studies by positive psychologists attempting to identify the key habits of happy people consistently note that a well-developed sense of gratitude is a key common trait. Expressing gratitude to other people has been found to be even more beneficial. A study by psychologist Martin Seligman at the University of Pennsylvania, USA, of a range of positive interventions, found that writing and delivering a letter of gratitude to a person who had never properly been thanked delivered the biggest and longest-lasting mood boost.

Keep a notebook

You don't need to devote much time to this; even noting down a few key moments from your day is beneficial. Take care not to dwell too much on negative experiences: a study comparing people who were encouraged to keep a gratitude diary to those encouraged to log their irritations found that those intent on noticing positive, rather than negative, experiences reported feeling significantly happier at the end of the process.[12] Having said that, other research shows that journalling after a traumatic experience, such as an operation, can boost recovery, so there is something in the cathartic expression of difficult feelings through writing, but only if they are left on the page and not used to reinforce your experiences.

Prioritise sleep

When sleep is compromised, our brains suffer. Insufficient, or poor-quality sleep reduces reaction speed and alertness – making it dangerous to drive, for example. There are reports of sleep-deprived people who have gone mad. Research also tells us that, over time, a sleep deficit increases the rate of cognitive decline,[13] and poor sleep quality can result in an increase of the protein deposits in the brain that lead to Alzheimer's disease.[14] On top of that you're also more likely to become depressed and experience 'brain fog'. And whilst poor sleep is often a symptom rather than a cause (because some other aspect of your well-being is interfering with your ability to get the rest you need), it often works the other way too, with poor sleep triggering or exacerbating a range of mental and physical symptoms.

Inadequate sleep impacts on the production of melatonin, the sleep hormone that regulates your sleep–wake rhythm. As a general rule, seven to seven and a half hours of sleep is optimal. A study of more than 9,000 people found that those who had either less than six or more than eight hours sleep had reduced memory function and decision-making ability. Insufficient sleep can also have serious genetic repercussions on your brain. Recent research compared the gene expression of a group of volunteers sleeping six hours a night for a week with that of a group who slept for eight hours a night. Even in that short time they observed that in those who had only six hours sleep, the normal function of 711 genes was distorted and approximately half of those, the genes associated with stress, tumour growth and inflammation, had increased their activity. In another experiment, the US General Services Administration found that employees who were exposed to more daylight, particularly in the morning, took less time to fall asleep at night, slept longer, and reported better moods. Workers who saw more light between 8am and 12pm, slept 20 minutes longer and took just 18 minutes on average to fall asleep – compared to their colleagues' 45 minutes.

In contrasting studies from New York University School of Medicine, researchers described the way sleep benefits the brain. They showed that sleep helps learning retention by encouraging the growth of 'dendritic spines' – mushroom-shaped protrusions that grow out of the ends of synapses, and help to connect brain cells and encourage communication of information across synapses.[15] While you sleep, the cerebrospinal fluid (CSF) in your brain pumps faster, flushing out the debilitating build-up of waste proteins that accumulate between brain cells when you are awake – and this includes the build-up of beta amyloid, the plaque-forming substance connected to Alzheimer's.[16] If waste is not properly flushed through, it accumulates as toxins, which in part accounts for the sluggish feelings you experience when, after a bad night's sleep, it's difficult to get your brain working and attention focused.

Action plan

- **Set yourself a regular sleep timetable** Go to bed and wake up at the same time every day – including weekends and holidays.

- **Keep your room temperature cool** Your body sleeps better when it's cooler – 18°C (65°F) is optimal.

- **Avoid caffeine after midday** Caffeine stays in your system long after you have consumed it and having a coffee late afternoon could make it harder to drop off at bedtime.

- **Don't look at any tech within two hours of going sleep** This includes phones, tablets and the TV before you go to sleep. Don't have them in your bedroom. The blue light from screens interferes with melatonin production, and a prolonged bout of screen-time before bed makes it harder to drop off.

- **Put a few drops of lavender oil on your pillow** A 2017 study showed that inhaling lavender oil significantly improved sleep quality and reduced anxiety levels of recovering coronary patients in a hospital setting.[17]

- **Make your bedroom as calm as possible** Remove all distractions from the bedroom to give your brain the best chance of disconnecting and recuperating. Don't store work papers in the room or have your computer visible.

- **Keep the room as dark as possible** Remove any distracting lights, consider black-out blinds if necessary. Light is for day and activity, dark is for night and sleep and, however small and dim, light confuses the brain. If you have to go to the bathroom during the night, try to do so without having to switch any lights on – it makes it much easier to go back to sleep as cortisol will not have been triggered. If, for safety, some light is necessary, have a very low-intensity light that plugs into a wall socket and, if possible, position it so that the light can't be seen from your bedroom.

➡ **Read my book** A full list of top sleep tips can be found in my book, *Reboot your Sleep: How to get a good night's rest*, available on Amazon.co.uk.

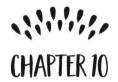

CHAPTER 10

COMPLEMENTARY THERAPIES THAT BOOST YOUR BRAIN

'By making us feel supported, by summoning the power of expectations and belief, by relaxing our bodies and reducing stress, mind-body therapies move molecules in our brains in a way that can reduce the ills we feel in our bodies.'

MELANIE WARNER, SCIENCE AND HEALTH AUTHOR

Just as we are all acutely aware of the fundamental necessities of eating and exercising well to help us reach a healthier, happier older age, regular focused 'brain care' can support your brain function and mental health alongside the lifestyle changes you make.

Optimising your brain function and mental health is a lifelong quest and there is always more that you can do. Where conventional medicine stops short of providing the direction you need, there are myriad complementary therapies to try. Not all of them will be appropriate, or effective, for your brain and emotional condition. But to help you navigate the dizzying variety of treatments on offer, and work out what might suit (and what might be worth skipping), here is the low-down on brain-specific treatments to try.

A-Z of therapies that calm, restructure and rewire your brain

The use of complementary and alternative approaches as an adjunct to conventional medical care is growing across the world. Certain therapies have been scientifically proven to affect the brain positively, changing physical structure and, in some cases, releasing the mental and emotional trauma that reduces brain function, but some have not. The information can be confusing, making it hard to separate the real from the junk science. Contradictory reviews abound on the internet, which makes for a chaotic minefield of information and misinformation.

To complicate things even further, complementary and alternative medicine (CAM) has little budget for expensive scientific research projects, while for the big pharmaceutical companies, many effective treatments offer insufficient profit margins to justify further investigation. As a result, some of the therapies here don't have solid research yet. But don't dismiss them out of hand. Anecdotal evidence shows that many are highly effective and all good science starts from good observation and telling a story about what has been seen, before then conducting further experiments; so never ignore 'anecdotal'.

The descriptions here are presented as an introduction to the therapy, and you won't be able to judge for yourself until you have experienced a specific therapy. Never take anyone else's opinion blindly as fact. Try them for yourself, one at a time, until you work out what's right for your brain, and your emotional condition. Only by trialling them yourself can you analyse the efficacy of any particular therapy on your own issues and tissues, and in every case, much depends on the skill and training of your particular therapist.

Acupuncture

Acupuncture can strengthen the physical structures of the brain because it improves both blood circulation and energy flow. For relief of mental stress, the key to acupuncture healing is via boosting what the Chinese describe as 'Shen', or the vital force and energetic flow of our system. If your Shen is low, Chinese medical practitioners believe you may well present with depression. The Shen Men, or 'Spirit Gate', is the most important point for brain/emotion/spirit balance. A series of acupuncture sessions will balance your energy flow, increasing the levels of Shen in your brain, boosting overall function, memory and focus. Acupuncture points stimulated by laser light have been shown to be as effective as needling and research demonstrates that the colour violet in particular stimulates energy circulation in the brain.[1]

Ear acupuncture

This is another way of boosting brain function as there are points in the ear that relate specifically to the brain stem, hippocampus, frontal cortex, and pineal and pituitary glands, which affect cognitive function. There are also points that affect aggression, psychosomatic reaction and depression. Key points can be seen below. You can also stimulate energy flow and improve symptoms simply by rubbing hard on the specific areas relating to your concerns, a few times daily. Rubbing the outer ridge immediately above the entrance to the ear canal stimulates activity in the vagus nerve, which connects head, heart and gut.

Key ear acupuncture points for the brain

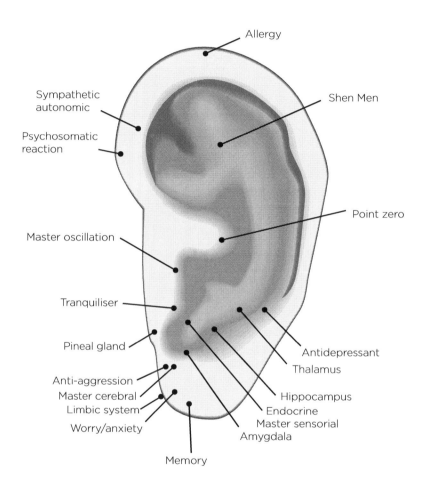

Amygdala point for modulating emotional processing, and calming fear responses.

Endocrine point calms hypersensitivity and balances endocrine hormones.

Hippocampus point for reducing neuron loss in the hippocampus, slowing cognitive impairment and memory loss.

Limbic system point for balancing emotion and formation of memories, and motivation of long-term memory and sense of smell.

Master cerebral point for boosting decision making and deep sleep. Reduces levels of anxiety, fear, worry, irritability, lack of concentration and anxiety. Used for obsessive compulsive disorder (OCD).

Master oscillation point for balancing right and left sides of the brain.

Master sensorial point sharpens blurred vision. Also affects tinnitus.

Shen Men calms the mind, alleviates stress, pain and tension. Reduces anxiety, depression and insomnia. Stimulates sluggish thinking.

Pineal gland point for regulating sleep and hormone production.

Point zero for overall brain balance. It also balances hormones.

Psychosomatic reaction point for calming disorders which involve both mind and body and lowers stress levels.

Sympathetic autonomic point reduces stress and balances the sympathetic/parasympathetic nervous system. Boosts blood circulation.

Thalamus point calms overexcitement and shock.

Tranquiliser point for reducing anxiety.

Chiropractic and osteopathy

Brain electroencephalography (EEG) scans show that chiropractic and osteopathic adjustments can change brain function. It is not merely the bones of the spine that are manipulated during a session; both therapies address your nerves too. By balancing any issues relating to the autonomic nervous system, osteopathy and chiropractic appear to rebalance the brain and adjust the flow of both the cerebrospinal fluid and the lymphatic system, boosting your overall immunity. An out-of-alignment atlas bone (the first cervical vertebra – C1), for instance, can constrict blood flow to the brain by up to 70 per cent (see Chapter 4 for more on this subject). Studies using fMRI showed changes in connections between the left and right sides of the brain directly after manipulation.[2]

Studies have demonstrated that the state of your spine is clearly linked to your thoughts, feelings and behaviours, and that back pain itself overloads the brain, which leads to difficulty concentrating and making decisions. The health of your spine has been linked to the health of your brain by the discovery of a thinning of the dorso-lateral prefrontal cortex in patients with back issues. Research now shows that not only does treating back pain halt this thinning, but it also reverses it.[3]

Research also shows that most chronic back pain isn't necessarily the result of injury, but can be caused by thoughts and feelings. So complementary therapies that shift psychological patterns can also shift both physical pain and emotional symptoms. Cognitive behavioural therapy (CBT) and mindfulness are the two most quoted therapies,[4] but emotional freedom technique (EFT) and eye movement desensitisation and reprocessing (EMDR) also address mental issues effectively, see opposite.

Cognitive behavioural therapy (CBT)

CBT looks at how your thoughts and beliefs affect your feelings and your behaviour and gives you tools to change your behaviour by altering your self-limiting thoughts. It helps you see that thoughts and feelings you have habitually, for whatever reason, taken as truths, may in fact be neither fact nor truth and are often influenced by the way you interpreted a certain situation at the time. Your therapist will look at why you think a certain way, and why, in doing so, you repeatedly reach a negative conclusion and will offer you other possibilities to put in its place instead. Six sessions are considered sufficient to change your patterns.

Recent studies now show, through observing brain scans, that CBT changes neuronal pathways in the brain. Research into patients with anxiety disorders[5] – including OCD, phobias, panic attacks and post-traumatic stress disorder (PTSD) – showed that CBT effectively modified dysfunctional neural activity through changes to the amygdala, hippocampus and cortical areas of the brain.

Craniosacral therapy

Cerebrospinal fluid (CSF) is the liquid that flows throughout the hollow spaces around your brain and spinal cord. It removes toxins stored in the tissues, delivers nutrients, and controls and cools the temperature of your brain, while also cushioning it from damage.

Blockages in the flow of CSF are thought by craniosacral therapists to contribute to certain neurological health issues, including autism and cerebral palsy, dyslexia and learning difficulties, depression, anxiety, epilepsy, and hormonal imbalances. Similarly, concussion, head, neck and temporomandibular joint (between the jaw and the skull) problems, spinal cord injuries, and types of dementia, are thought to be linked to the flow of CSF.

Craniosacral therapy uses gentle pressure around the cranial bones of the skull to release constrictions and lightly pump the CSF, relieving any compression in the head, neck and nerves. This normalises the function of the entire central nervous system and boosts the immune system in the process.[6] Craniosacral therapy also calms the central nervous system, moving you out of a constantly stressed state, and lowering adrenaline levels.

Craniosacral therapy and tinnitus

Evidence shows that craniosacral therapy has some success with tinnitus. At the root of tinnitus there is likely to be some sort of inflammation in your inner ear. This increases the quantity of lymphatic fluid in the area, which causes pressure to build up and block normal circulation. If you can identify what has caused that initial inflammation and reverse the problem, often the tinnitus disappears. A session with a craniosacral therapist will rebalance the flow of CSF, releasing energy blockages in the area, so desensitising your hearing and alleviating symptoms. Therapists work gently with the CSF inside your skull, manipulating the different bones around your brain, and releasing and balancing any pressure that may be affecting your auditory nerve.

Emotional freedom technique (EFT)

Also known as 'tapping', this is a technique that is used by some counsellors, therapists and hypnotherapy practitioners. It fuses affirmations with 'tapping' on acupressure points, and advocates recommend it for a wide range of psychological issues, from depression to fatigue and low self-esteem.[7] Gary Craig, the founder of EFT, carried out research which demonstrated that this technique was effective for healing traumatic brain injury.[8]

An hour-long session of EFT has been shown to reduce levels of cortisol – your stress hormone – by 24 per cent.[9]

Eye movement desensitisation and reprocessing (EMDR)

A technique that combines eye movement, hand tapping and auditory beats with the controlled re-imagining of past trauma, EMDR, has been approved by the World Health Organisation (WHO) and the UK's National Institute for Clinical Excellence (NICE) as an effective treatment for PTSD. Developed in the late 80s by American clinical psychologist Francine Shapiro, EMDR is based around the principle that if a person recalls the worst aspect of a trauma, along with its associated physical symptoms, and is simultaneously instructed to move their eyes from side to side, it helps them to reprocess the memory in a controlled way, desensitising the person to the trauma and reprogramming their brain.[10] The recent availability of EMDR applications that you can download onto a tablet or smart phone now makes the therapy accessible as a daily stress-release practice at home.

Hypnotherapy

Hypnotherapy is an effective tool for clearing trauma and stress, as it rapidly releases associations between specific issues and the events or emotions that triggered it. An experienced practitioner will put you into a state of deep relaxation where you remain acutely awake and conscious of everything around you. At the same time, your mind and body sink into a deeply focused state that enables the therapist to access and change deep habitual patterns in your non-conscious brain. They can make verbal suggestions to you in order to help transform aspects of your behaviour, releasing anxieties, fears or phobias simply and effectively.[11]

Intravenous therapy

Also known as IV therapy, this is a treatment where a bag of carefully combined liquid nutrients, usually hanging on a tall metal stand, slowly drips its contents through a clear plastic tube into a canula inserted into a vein in your hand or arm. The nutrients pass directly into your bloodstream, where they are circulated and used where they are needed by the body, by-passing the gastric juices that so often destroy up to 85 per cent of the benefits of vitamins and minerals when you swallow them with a glass of water; with intravenous therapy 100 per cent of the nutrients go directly into your bloodstream.

However, IV therapy is controversial. Lack of regulation means that beauticians can offer it as a treatment, which is a concern as there is the potential to disturb your electrolyte balance if the infusion rate is not carefully monitored. In extreme cases, this could cause swelling in the brain, or heart failure. The fluids also contain a lot of salt, which can make them inadvisable for anybody with high blood pressure.

Only try this treatment if you have read up on it thoroughly, and always go to a reputable clinic, as many qualified medical practitioners offer medical-grade treatment. There are a number of brain specific infusions.

IV combinations

Myers' cocktail This is a mineral and vitamin mixture that forms the base of many treatments. It includes essential vitamins and trace minerals – vitamin C, the B vitamins (B1, 2, 3, 5, 6, 9 [folic acid] and 12) and magnesium. You can ask for advice on specific add-ons for a targeted brain booster.

Hydrogen peroxide Your cells need oxygen to survive and carry out their daily tasks. This treatment increases oxygen levels, so helping to repair the body's tissues and boost white blood cells, as well as reducing the plaque that builds up on the artery walls, and wiping out bacteria and viruses.

Magnesium EDTA Removes calcification or plaque build-up in the arteries and has been found to reduce brain inflammation.

Glutathione As we age, our levels of glutathione, a substance comprised of three amino acids made by the liver, reduces by around 10 per cent every decade. Known as the 'master antioxidant' it wipes out free radicals, increasing energy levels and improving brain function, boosts immunity, detoxifies the liver and reduces inflammation. Replacing it intravenously is an effective health tool and it has been used to treat Alzheimer's, Parkinson's, Huntington's, and Lyme diseases, as well as cancer, cystic fibrosis, and multiple sclerosis.

Silver hydrosol This is nano-sized particles of pure colloidal silver suspended in water. An antimicrobial substance, silver hydrosol is used to treat bacterial, fungal and viral infections in health clinics in the USA, but is less widely known in the UK. It has been used with some success in the treatment of Lyme disease.

Vitamin B12 (methylcobalamin) Many people are deficient in B12, which is needed for many of the body's functions, in particular it speeds metabolism and boosts energy levels. It is found in high concentrations in the soil that animals graze on, but over-farming means that the soil in which mass-produced fruit and vegetables are grown is itself depleted of B12. Given intravenously, B12 passes through the blood–brain barrier and gets directly to the brain. There are several types of B12, though, so make sure you read the labels carefully. Cyanocobalamin, a synthetic form of B12 that doesn't absorb well, is found in most of the supplements you buy across the counter because it is less expensive and more stable to manufacture. Methylcobalamin is the form of B12 you need as it is more efficiently absorbed by the body tissues, the brain and the nervous system. Methylcobalamin has been shown to relieve symptoms of multiple sclerosis, Parkinson's and Alzheimer's diseases and, in high doses, boosts brain neurons and nerve regeneration.[12]

Thiamine (B1) Essential for healthy brain and body function, B1 allows the body to convert carbohydrates into energy. Deficiency is common and low levels can lead to symptoms of poor blood sugar control and diabetes, cognitive decline, memory loss, fatigue and neuropathy.

Intravenous treatments for heavy metal removal

The administration of special drugs that bind to metals in your blood so that they can be excreted from your body through the kidneys and urine, or chelation therapy, has been used to treat metal poisoning for many years. Toxic metals such as mercury, copper, aluminium and cadmium, are lethal to the health of the human body. If your levels are high, your brain is likely to be compromised, and one of the quickest ways to improve your health is to remove them from your body. But it should only be administered by a qualified medical practitioner to prevent overloading the body's elimination systems.

Calcium EDTA binds to heavy metals, particularly lead.

DMPS (a sulfonic acid chelating agent that has an impossibly long name – look it up on the internet) binds to heavy metals, particularly to mercury.

Phosphatidylcholine, another binding agent, is hard to find, but is one of the most effective toxic metal chelation therapies.

Kinesiology (or muscle testing)

Your brain captures everything that has ever happened to you, from the moment you were conceived, recording the emotions that accompanied each and every event. The chemicals that are the biology of emotions become part of the cells of your body and brain in what is often, in energy medicine, referred to as 'cellular memory'. Kinesiology works to release the feelings that may be causing, consciously or non-consciously, problems for you in your everyday life. It gets a bad rap in the scientific press. But I'm a firm believer in it, because I've seen it work. I'm a trained kinesiologist, and have watched numerous people overcome emotional and physical problems through its use.

Kinesiology uses the 'language' of your body – emotions, and the complexity of feelings they create, which are locked into the neurochemistry of your cells – to interpret the messages your body is sending to you. Many of us struggle to hear what our bodies are saying because there is so much 'noise' in the way. The giant suitcases of emotional baggage we haul around with us are filled with the continuing difficulties of the past. When your inner space is filled to the brim with painful 'stuff', it not only leaves little room for relevant emotions in the present, but it also interferes with your ability to appreciate what is going on at a deep level.

This therapy cuts through the noise, delving deep into your non-conscious self to release the pain, restoring physical and mental effectiveness in the process. The therapist will use muscle testing to identify problems or blockages. Typically, weeks afterwards, you will notice that something that had been constantly in your thoughts, perhaps for years, is no longer invading as once it did. Once dealt with, those thoughts and feelings never return with the power they previously had.

Types of kinesiology

Health kinesiology This is a branch of muscle testing that is particularly focused on the brain. Certain techniques that have been developed can re-wire the brain's habitual pathways, facilitating change in thinking and feeling. Health kinesiology removes any blockages in the meridian and energy pathways of your body and brain and helps you to think more clearly, improving your ability to evaluate, solve problems, think creatively and think laterally.[13]

One-brain kinesiology This is a powerful branch of kinesiology that enables you to identify specific unresolved issues and then helps you to override the messaging in your conscious brain. One-brain kinesiology allows you to access your old behavioural and emotional patterns, giving you the tools to disconnect from them and reprogramme your non-conscious mind's present day messaging. Sessions gently release trauma and mental patterns that may be holding you back, creating remarkable life-changing shifts.

Psych-K This is another efficient way to release the control that subliminal programming has on your day-to-day thoughts, feelings and emotions. It has been written about extensively by American biologist, Bruce Lipton, in books such as his *The Biology of Belief*, www.psych-k.com.

Oxygen therapy

Your brain needs three times as much oxygen as your muscles to function efficiently.[14] If it becomes oxygen-starved, it simply stops functioning properly. Few of us nowadays breathe as regularly as we should, with the deep diaphragmatic breaths that carry air and oxygen into the blood and on to the brain. Many of us breathe through our mouths rather than our noses, which further reduces the amount of oxygen that ultimately reaches the brain cells.

Oxygen therapy can provide a fast-acting pick-me-up that boosts your brain function.

In a pressurised hyperbaric oxygen chamber your body is subjected to the same force that it would experience 3.6m (11ft) under water. This pressure forces you to breathe in 95 per cent pure oxygen, rapidly oxygenating your body and brain – and the oxygen remains in your bloodstream for several weeks after treatment. Hyperbaric therapy has been shown to relieve depression and multiple sclerosis and help after brain injury or a stroke. It has a positive effect on symptoms of Alzheimer's and Parkinson's diseases.

Far-infrared (FIR) oxygen domes, which raise your body temperature and deliver pure oxygen, are another option. The infrared heat warms your body to above 37˚C (98.6˚F), increasing your core temperature. This stimulates your natural killer (NK) cells, boosts the immune system, and increases blood flow to the area heated. FIR heat combined with oxygen expands the blood vessels, unloading toxins, reducing inflammation and relieving tension at the same time as rebooting the brain.

Tai Chi

Also known as tai chi chuan, this combines deep breathing, relaxation and flowing movements and boosts your ability to judge where your body sits in space – an attribute that declines with age. Regular practice of even an hour a week (at home or in a group) will strengthen the neural pathways in the brain that sustain balance.

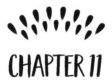

CHAPTER 11

MACHINES THAT STIMULATE YOUR BRAIN

*'I'm interested in things that change the world
or that affect the future and wondrous, new
technology where you see it, and you're like,
"Wow, how did that even happen?"'*

ELON MUSK, TECHNOLOGY ENTREPRENEUR AND ENGINEER

There are a multitude of brain-boosting machines that use wave frequencies of colour, light and/or sound to change your cognition for the better to help your brain stay younger than its years. And as technology improves, so will they.

It is becoming clearer and clearer that human beings are not, in fact, as we have thought for the past 120 years, psychological systems, but they are *energy* systems. And it is energy, in the form of light, sound, vibration and electricity that our brains respond to. Neuroscience provides evidential back-up that these interventions can really change the physical structure of the brain. They aren't placebo, or perception effects – they directly affect the brain. The discovery of neuroplasticity – the ever-changing structure of the brain's pathways – makes the phrase 'use it or lose' it more appropriate than ever. You may exercise your body regularly, but it's more and more clear that you need to exercise your brain as often. Science has confirmed that your brain grows new brain cells daily, whatever your age, so the possibilities are very much greater than had been thought, even quite recently.

What follows is a selection of brain-therapy machines that I have tried myself and found effective – many of which you can buy for home use. I have divided them into four sections; some work with light, others with colour, sound or magnetic fields and electricity. Many of them combine two or more approaches.

How can you tell how well your brain is working?

Advances in neuroimaging techniques in the last 30 years reveal the brain as never before. It is possible to see which parts of the brain become active, or 'light up', in the presence of specific emotions and measure the electricity generated by neurons in different situations. Scientists can even calculate the changes that a stressful experience will have on specific structures in the brain. A 2016 study confirmed that electromagnetic waves, particularly colour and sound, affect neural cells according to their vibration.[1] Specific wave frequencies can strengthen your neurons, increase your attention span and calm inflammation, alongside boosting your memory and stimulating new nerve cells and synapses.

So which scanner is good for what?

X-ray imaging These can show the physical structures in your brain, but not how they work with their changing electrical processes.

continued...

Functional magnetic resonance imaging (fMRI) This form of MRI can show when nerve cells are active because oxygen circulation increases as cells become more active. It shows which structure in the brain is active at any given time, and how that area's activity level changes over a period of time. This enables us to link neural pathways and brain structures to mental or emotional processes. Scientists can even examine 'slices', or sections of your brain, as if it was dissected in a lab. Check out the Obelab Nirsit scanner, obelab.com.

The eVox system Developed by Evoke neuroscience, this is an US FDA-approved device that offers different brain function tests. Done over a period of 25 minutes it can give a clear map of where any dysfunction may be occurring. It measures various factors:

- Cognitive response measurements work out how quickly and consistently your brain signals your muscles to react.

- Brain speed tests measure how efficiently your brain can acquire new visual and auditory information.

- Heart rate variability (HRV) assesses how well your body tolerates physical and psychological stress by measuring the balance between the sympathetic and parasympathetic systems.

- Neuro imaging measures the electrical activity on the surface of the brain, creating a map of the area. You have to wear a cap for this one!

EEG (electroencephalography) neurofeedback systems

Brain pathways become stronger the more often the same neural networks are used. Neurofeedback systems map your brain and collect data on how the electrophysiology that creates your mind is working. This shows you where you struggle emotionally and teaches you how to shift your habitual pathways. Moving from one dominating brainwave to another raises your frequencies and improves aspects of your thinking. EEG neurofeedback gives you the opportunity to teach your brain how to break away from involuntary negative habits and get back to a neutral unstressed state.

A set of sensors is fixed to something that looks like a swimming cap, which will effectively 'listen' to and record, on a printed trace-out, the electrical wave impulses from your brain, so creating a detailed map of your brain activity. With the cap in place you sit comfortably in a chair, while the neurofeedback machine plays a video, a game or music intended to re-train your brain and feeds back to you when your brain is meeting its training target and when it is not, allowing you to move your brain into different and eventually better and healthier ways.

Different brain-wave frequencies are linked to different mental states and disorders. Alpha-wave biofeedback, for example, has been shown to be a useful tool for treating anxiety and depression. Research shows that by learning to relax out of a habitual stress response, levels of anxiety decrease.

If you suffer from attention deficit disorder (ADD) your brain is likely to show high levels of low-frequency theta waves. Similarly, if you have suffered traumatic brain injuries, theta waves will dominate.

Light machines

Modern medicine is increasingly using light for healing. Light is powerful and without sufficient light your brain simply does not function optimally. Light photons are taken in through your skin, and travel along neural pathways and your spinal cord until they reach the brain, re-invigorating brain cells and boosting hormones. Applying light to the head has a positive effect on physical and emotional neurological issues and has been shown to help symptoms for conditions as far ranging as depression, chemo-brain, and Parkinson's disease, improving both memory and mood. Full-spectrum light boxes have been developed to reduce the overwhelming winter blues that trigger seasonal affective disorder (SAD). Ultraviolet light treats the brain to help with sleep problems. Laser lights can be used for acupuncture instead of needles, and low-level lasers have been found to be effective for chronic and acute pain and inflammation in the brain.

But the 'right' type of light is crucial – light can heal, but it can also harm. Bright, harsh lights can enhance aggression. The blue light from your smart phone or tablet screens stimulates the brain, disturbing circadian rhythms, interfering with production of the sleep hormone melatonin and making it hard to sleep at night. Too much light in a room can make people close up, and restrain conversation and communication. Conversely, too little light makes people nervous and, again, affects communication adversely. Like the three bears and their porridge, light levels need to be just right.

The wavelengths and frequencies of light, both visible and invisible, are the key to many types of healing and different types can have different effects.

220

Far-infrared (FIR) light This generates heat and is used in saunas to detox from toxic metals that may affect your brain.

Near-infrared light (NIR) This therapy positively affects the eyes, muscles, nerves, skin and immune system and has been shown to improve mental reaction time and performance.

Pulsing light-emitting diodes (LEDs) Every tissue and cell in the body absorbs and reacts to a specific wavelength of light, so pulsing LEDs that use a single frequency, or specific colour, have been developed to cover the entire spectrum. Using only a single frequency or colour, practitioners can heal different health problems and this treatment has been found to be helpful to patients after a stroke, concussion and internal problems in the brain[2] (see box below). LED light can penetrate up to 20cm (8in), so can successfully reach the brain through the skull. Light shone on to the back of neck stimulates brain cells, in particular the occipital cortex area of the brain.

The brain benefits of colour healing

Research studies have shown that the colours you surround yourself with have an impact on your physical and emotional health.[3] As much as 60 per cent of your mood and reaction to events will be down to the colour of your surroundings. What's more, different shades of those colours adjust your heart rate and blood pressure accordingly.[4]

Red The most powerful colour in the spectrum, red can boost poor circulation. It increases mental alertness, raises emotional awareness, and activates the pituitary hormones. The wavelengths of red light lower inflammation and boost mood, stimulating pain-reducing neurotransmitters (endorphins and enkephalins). Cancer should never be treated with red light as it stimulates cells to grow.

continued...

Orange An anti-depressant that inspires creative thinking, orange stimulates the immune system.

Yellow A colour that strengthens the nerves and the mind, yellow elevates the psyche and spirit, speeds digestion and benefits the liver, lymph and stomach. Yellow also lowers inflammation whilst boosting circulation, helps mental concentration and relieves depression.

Green This is soothing to both mind and body. It balances hormonal issues, strengthens the nervous system and increases immunity. Green also strengthens against panic attacks and addictions.

Turquoise Cool, calming and soothing, turquoise is good for the nervous system and calms inflammation.

Blue The most calming and relaxing of all the colours, blue reduces anxiety and blood pressure, calms the nerves and cools inflammation.

Indigo Calms the nervous system and is anti-inflammatory. Improves sleep.

Violet Soothes mental stress, can help treat depression and balances the pineal and pituitary glands. Leonardo da Vinci said that he could increase the power of meditation 10 times by sitting under a violet ray emitted by the stained-glass windows of a church.

Did you know?

We, like the plants, are light-activated beings. Our cells are energised and powered by light, so need it to survive. Placing an LED light on your belly button, which sits in front of the abdominal aorta (the largest artery in the body), will flood light into your whole blood system.[5] In the space of 20 minutes every drop of blood in the body passes in front of the light, which increases the activity of your white and red blood cells, B-cells and T-cells, boosting your immune system as well as your brain.

Light on the back of the neck can have a positive effect on your vision. It triggers the occipital cortex area of the brain, stimulating more than 20 billion neurons and boosting the mitochondria that produce the energy needed to optimise your mental function.[6]

Photobiomodulation (PBM)

This is a form of light therapy that uses LEDs or low-level cold lasers to beam near NIR and red light waves into the brain. These light frequencies pass easily through the skull and re-energise the mitochondria, the energy batteries of the brain cells, preventing existing neurons from dying. This repairs any damage and triggers the birth of new neurons. Research has found that PBM increases electricity levels and blood flow as well as reducing inflammation in the brain and increasing the production and activity of neurotransmitters.[7]

Studies now show that beaming a cold laser onto the brain can improve function in the frontal cortex, boosting memory and the ability to focus. Other research suggests that stimulating different brain regions with infrared light should affect different brain functions.[8] Cold lasers work by using energy that boosts alpha-wave frequency in the brain and have been shown to boost ATP production (the primary energy source of our cells) by as much as 150 per cent. The lasers can be used to stimulate the points in the ear that trigger the release of endorphins and the neurotransmitters dopamine, serotonin and oxytocin.[9]

The Vielight 810 infrared and Vielight Neuro

This is a brain PBM device that gently infuses the blood and brain with NIR photons through short 25-minute, daily sessions. It clips onto the side of your nose and beams light up inside it, directing it into the deep, usually inaccessible, areas of your brain. Inside your nose there is minimal hair and thin skin, as well as a dense concentration of blood vessels close to the surface, so light energy can enter easily and effectively.

The Vielight 810 uses NIR light on an 810nm wavelength, and pulses at 10Hz, which researchers have found repairs cells, neurons and neural networks. The wavelength and strength of its pulsing programme sends photons deep into the brain's ventral areas where dopamine, which controls sleep regulation, is made. Boost your ventral neurons and you balance your ability to sleep long and deeply. NIR energy also helps release serotonin, the calming neurotransmitter that has been found to play a part in sleep cycles. Serotonin is needed by the pineal gland to make melatonin, the hormone that is connected to healthy sleep. Low serotonin levels lead to sleep disruption and insomnia. Using the Vielight 810 regularly resets your circadian rhythms and users report deeper sleep and more energy on waking.

The Neuro, a metal device with micro-chip boosted LED diodes attached, fits closely to your head and offers serious hope for improvement of a range of brain issues. It beams near-infrared light through various points on your skull and your forehead, penetrating deep into your brain, increasing both neuroplasticity and oxygenation. Regular use has been shown to positively affect depression and anxiety and research demonstrates significant improvement in symptoms in cases of dementia. Combine the two machines and you simultaneously stimulate both the ventral and cortical brain areas.[10]

www.vielight.com

SOTA Lightworks

The LightWorks comes with a paddle; one side containing 60 high intensity red LED lights emitting a wavelength of 660 nanometers (nm) and a light output of 718 milliwatts (mW) and the other 57 near infrared LED lights with an 850 nm wavelength and 455 mW light output. Additional paddles are available with yellow/orange and blue/green light combinations.

www.cytodoc.com

The Yumalite

One in three people in the UK are affected by depression and the winter blues, known as seasonal affective disorder (SAD) syndrome – women more frequently than men – and in the USA up to 20 per cent of the population suffer from it. Lack of light plays a part, and the further north you live and the less sunshine you are exposed to, the greater the problem. Putting the light back in your life so to speak, re-jigs your brain and your mood along with it. The Yumalite is a small and light device, sold by a Canadian health company, SOTA Instruments. It attaches to your head and beams white or red LEDs into your eyes; you can wear it and walk around the house, getting on with your normal day. Its light frequencies penetrate deep into your brain, regulating your circadian rhythms and stimulating melatonin. The red light also helps balance exposure to an overload of the blue rays given off by our computers, tablets and smart phones.

www.cytodoc.com

Sound machines

By working with your brain waves you have the potential to heal your body and mind because our bodies respond to the specific frequencies of our brain waves which can trigger cell repair and regeneration. Theta and delta waves represent the non-conscious mind: add more delta and you feel at one with the Universe; add more theta and you have the potential for healing. Beta and gamma waves represent the conscious mind, and alpha provides the bridge between the two groups. Up your alpha levels and your conscious and non-conscious minds start talking.

Stimulating the brain with gamma waves helps stimulate the hippocampus and the newly discovered region of the brain called the retrosplenial cortex, the areas of the brain directly associated with perception, memory and navigation.[11]

Which brain wave does what?

Sound waves operate at different frequencies: hertz, or Hz, describes the frequency of sound.

Delta waves 0–4 Hz

Delta are the slowest brain waves and are typically experienced in deep dreamless sleep – a state that allows the brain to stop producing beta-amyloid and instead reduce any build-up of plaques.[12] When your brain is producing delta waves you may experience a feeling of merging with the infinite, you lose awareness of the everyday world and feel an all-encompassing oneness with the Universe. The brains of intuitives and meditators have higher than normal levels of delta waves. Delta waves stimulate growth hormone production, and enhance memory and learning.

continued...

This is the wave experienced when you are creating, losing all awareness of the outer world and is the state where inner healing is thought to occur.[13]

- 0.16Hz increases activity in the synaptic connections between neurons in the hippocampus.[14]

- 0.19 and 0.37Hz These are the only two frequencies that boost production of telomerase,[15] the enzyme that repairs the telomeres of your chromosomes. Longer telomeres are connected to a reduction of senescent cell numbers and are synonymous with a healthier and longer life.

- 0.5–3 Hz Stimulates regeneration of nerve cells.[16]

Theta waves 4–8Hz

This is the next slowest brain frequency – the one you experience when you are in shallow sleep. Theta is the wave used by all healers, of whatever belief system or practice, to heal. This is the frequency of rapid eye movement (REM). Memories of either good or bad emotional experiences can trigger theta waves.

- 5–10Hz Reduces lower back pain.[17]

- 6.4Hz Regenerates human cartilage cells[18] and increases levels of antioxidants, reducing the free radicals that cause ageing.

- 7.5–30Hz Enhances DNA repair – 9 Hz is the most effective frequency.[19]

Alpha waves 8–12Hz

This is a state of relaxed brain alertness. Time spent in alpha will boost your brain, improving mood, learning and memory and upping serotonin levels.[20]

continued...

- 10Hz Works on DNA[21] and reduces depression. It enables the neurons of the brain to take in more light to boost both neurons and the cells, and in doing so increases creativity.

- 4–12Hz Fires up the neurons in the hippocampus connected to memory and learning, particularly at 10Hz and above.[22]

Beta waves 13–25Hz

These waves are divided into two different ranges – high beta at 15–25Hz and low beta at 13–15Hz.

- 13–15Hz Low beta is generated when you are processing information and is indicative of a calm, focused state of mind. Associated with alertness and improved concentration.

- 15–25Hz High beta is the wave your brain clicks into when under great stress. It causes a rise in cortisol and adrenaline levels and ages your body more quickly. This is the so-called 'monkey mind' state where people with anxiety, frustration or high stress levels spend much of their time. It is also associated with feelings of blame, guilt, anger and fear.

Gamma waves 25–100 Hz

These are the brain waves associated with genius and flashes of inspiration and high gamma activity is linked to high IQ. Gamma is associated with raised levels of intellect and creativity – the feeling you get when you are 'in the zone'. It integrates and synchronises information from all the different areas of the brain,[23] and is the wave observed

continued...

in large flares when monks are asked to meditate on compassion.[24] It is also associated with improved memory retention, focused attention and data processing. Linking theta and gamma together improves memory still further, especially a detailed recall of the past.[25]

- 40Hz This is the specific frequency that is triggering hope for Alzheimer's disease. In a study that flashed 40Hz light into the brains of mice, it was observed that, within an hour of exposure, levels of beta amyloid reduced by 50 per cent.[26] This frequency increases the numbers of microglia – the cells that eat up dead cells, amyloid plaques and misshapen proteins.[27] It has been suggested that combining 10Hz and 40Hz may achieve even greater stimulation. This gamma wave is also thought to enhance memory cognition and information processing. In a study pending publication, gamma pulse rate at 40Hz has consistently and significantly up-regulated the higher oscillations of gamma, beta and alpha, and down-regulated theta and delta.

- 50Hz Increases production of stem cells.[28]

- 75Hz Triggers genes that produce anti-inflammatory proteins in the body.[29]

Binaural beat therapy

Re-aligning your brain by using specific frequencies can be a powerful tool for healing. Brain entrainment is a methodology whereby your brain naturally synchronises its frequencies to regular outside rhythms. Have you ever seen the YouTube video of the pendulum clocks, all ticking at different rates, which eventually synchronise by themselves? Or the metronomes, started at different times and ticking at different rates, that synchronise their sound and beat within the space of a minute?

When a single frequency is repeatedly played, all surrounding discordant frequencies in close range eventually align themselves until all are vibrating at the same beat. Musical pulse similarly synchronises the brain to its beat. Binaural beat is a type of sound therapy that has been shown to change brainwave patterns, and balance the right and left sides of the brain. Wearing a pair of headphones, your right and left ears listen to two different frequencies yet perceive it as a single tone or 'beat'. Specific sound combinations reboot different functions of your brain.

Binaural beat therapy has also been shown to boost the main hormones responsible for brain health moving into older age: affecting cortisol (which is linked to memory and learning), DHEA and melatonin, which improves the ability to sleep, giving the brain time to repair and revitalise. Try the myNoise or Atmosphere apps.

Cellular-aging expert Dr Vincent Giampapa carried out a study that showed that listening to binaural beats, four times a day for three days, raised DHEA levels by an average of 43.77 per cent, and melatonin levels between 97 and 300 per cent. Cortisol levels dropped by an average of 46 per cent, which reduces both stress and anxiety.

A word of caution, though, if you have serious heart problems or suffer from epilepsy, binaural beat therapy is not recommended.

LED 40Hz light and sound machines

Exposure to LED light or sound at 40Hz increases gamma brain waves, entraining the brain, boosting focus and activating the microglia, the cells that clean up beta amyloid plaques in the brain.[30] In mice, exposure to LED lights, to create higher levels of gamma waves, was found to decrease amyloid plaques, and so could potentially be an effective treatment for Alzheimer's disease. Flickering visible light at 40Hz stimulates the visual cortex and helps the brain to restore itself. Try out the Gamma Light audio entrainment device, or invest in one of their desktop lamps. www.gammalighttherapy.com

Machines for meditation

There are devices that can help you reach a relaxed state by lowering stress levels, or understand how effectively you meditate.

Nucalm

This is the world's first and only patented neuroscience technology proven to lower stress and improve your sleep quality without drugs. It flips the switch in your brain that moves you from a stressful state of high cortisol and adrenaline to one of deep relaxation. It slows down your mind, and restores balance to your autonomic nervous system, putting you into REM sleep, which is that state where the body begins to heal itself. Nucalm impacts the deep midbrain, temporal cortex, cerebellum and the brainstem. It has been scientifically shown to achieve the same deep meditative state experienced by monks who have been practising daily for 20 years or more – and all from using it for only 20 minutes a day.

Over a period of time, Nucalm will train your brain waves. It takes them from the beta range associated with normal everyday living (13–30Hz per second), or even from the high beta range waves associated with anxiety and fear (23–40Hz per second), and moves them into the alpha and theta ranges (4–12Hz per second) associated with deep relaxation. If you can get your brainwaves into the theta range, it is impossible to be anxious.

Nucalm consists of a headphone, which plays a series of calming music tracks designed to distract your conscious mind. Behind the music are a series of imprinted binaural beats that gradually bring your body into a state of deep relaxation. First, you rub a special gel (a patented Nucalm formula that includes GABA, the calming neurotransmitter) on either side of your neck. Then you attach two micro-current stimulation patches behind each ear, which relaxes you even further. Finally, you put on a light-blocking eye mask, then lie back and listen to a selection of soothing tracks of guitar and piano music and softly moving water.
www.nucalm.com

The Muse

Have you ever wondered whether you are meditating 'correctly'? Muse is a brain training tracker that makes you aware of how your brain is working and allows you to train it to remain in a calm state. It's a wearable headphone connected to an app that uses EEG (electroencephalography) to track the brain's electrical activity. Your mind state fluctuates, sometimes it is calm, and at other times active or even hyper-active. The Muse's brain-sensing technology shows you how to get to, and stay in, the calm mind place by changing the intensity of sounds that it plays to you as you meditate, by feeding you the sound of peaceful weather on a beach or in a rainforest. As your mind wanders off, the weather sounds get louder and louder, enabling you to switch your state, reverting to the calm and accessing the peaceful sounds once again as you do so. After a period of time, you automatically 'know' how to be in that zone. It has seven sensors, grouped into five different points – one behind each ear and three on the forehead. The App, which links to your phone, allows you to monitor your progress and see how often your attention wandered, or you moved or opened your eyes.
www.choosemuse.com

The Kasina

This is the ultimate mind relaxation machine, produced by MindPlace, a company that has been developing meditation technology since 1988. Their Kasina system is simple to use – and fun too. It looks like a smart phone, with a dial that gives you access to more than 50 different tracks. You don a wraparound 'ganzframe' pair of glasses that blanks out your surroundings and accompanies the specific frequencies of sound with a symphony of flashing LED lights that imprint colours into your open eyes, triggering deep relaxation.

The different light and sound frequencies trigger brainwave states, which stimulate your brain – effectively waking it up with a targeted concert of colours and sounds. The science shows that flooding your brain with specific frequencies can reduce your stress levels, release negative emotions and achieve a deeply relaxed, focused state similar to that achieved by meditation. www.kasina.co.uk

Vibration machines

TouchPoints uses bilateral alternating stimulation technology (BLAST) to restore calm in your brain and boost rational thinking. Touchpoints are two small devices that buzz and vibrate – at a different rate and timing – to override your brain's habitual patterns and in the process release any build-up of stress. Just by holding them in the palm of your hands – or wearing them on your wrists – has been shown to reduce stress levels by up to 70 per cent.

The devices have three settings, which you adjust according to the severity of your symptoms.

- Blue light triggers a calming beat and rhythm – useful if you are feeling overloaded by the day's workload or to-do list.

- Purple is for more extreme situations when anxiety and panic threaten to overwhelm you.

- Yellow helps you get to sleep at night; you'll be out like a light within minutes.

There is solid science behind the bilateral technology of TouchPoints. Remove the stress and your body simply starts functioning more efficiently. There are a multitude of research papers available online demonstrating the effectiveness of the technology. They all show remarkable results with heart rate, blood pressure levels, depression, anxiety and memory. They improve motor function in Parkinson's, and decrease symptoms of hyperactivity, ADHD and obsessive compulsive disorder (OCD).[31] www.thetouchpointsolution.com

Electric, or magnetic field, machines

It's all about electricity. Whether your brain works properly, or doesn't, may well be down to how efficiently your neurons and their receptors manage to move their signalling around your brain. Metaphorically speaking, if there's no electricity, the lights in your brain begin to sink into darkness. Put it back in, however, and your systems effectively light, or 'fire', up.

The PlatoWork headset

Now available for home use, this wearable transcranial direct current stimulation (tDCS) headset sends a weak electric current through specific areas of your brain to activate the neurons, boosting memory, concentration and focus. You need to wear it for 3 minutes daily for optimal benefit.
www.platoscience.com

The Halo

This is a brain-stimulating tDCS device that enables your brain to enter a similar state of hyperlearning capacity and knowledge integration that your brain was capable of when you were very young. It sends tiny electrical currents from electrodes attached to headphones into the brain, and within 20 minutes, boosts the motor cortex, enhancing mental skills, learning and concentration and reinforcing new neural pathways and muscle memory. www.haloneuro.com

Transcranial magnetic stimulation (TMS)

TMS uses short magnetic pulses, applied by magnetic coils with a field strength similar to that of an MRI (magnetic resonance imaging) machine, to create a low direct current that stimulates the brain's cortex. The machine analyses your brain's electrical activity to work out where the communication between your neurons is over or under active, then rebalances the flow of electricity. The use of TMS was approved by the US Food and Drug Administration (FDA) in 2008 and the UK's National Institute for Health and Care Excellence (NICE) approved its use in 2015, but it is only available privately. It is mainly used as a treatment for severe depression and anxiety.

Fifty per cent of patients find their symptoms significantly improved after a course of treatment and one in three experience complete relief of their symptoms. Sessions take between 20 and 40 minutes and need to be repeated five times a week for four to six weeks.[32]

Portable neuromodulation stimulator (PoNS)

Recent research suggests that one of the most effective ways of stimulating the brain may be via your tongue. The tongue contains more nerve endings and receptors than any other area of your body, and it provides direct access to the brainstem via pulses that affect two major cranial nerves. The PoNS machine uses gentle electrical currents to stimulate the tongue and boost – and reboot – the neurons of the spinal cord, the cortex, the cerebellum and the entire central nervous system. When neural networks are disrupted, the area of the body connected to the area of the brain that is no longer working optimally will also stop functioning. By stimulating the brain's neuroplasticity, however, any disrupted neuronal networks can be re-invigorated and damage reversed.[33]

Pulsed electromagnetic field (PEMF) machines

Research shows that if low-energy, PEMFs resonate in harmony with the Earth's magnetic field they can re-align the cells of the body, increasing energy production at a cellular level. PEMF machines differ from one another principally according to the strength of their magnetic field. The machine is connected to a full-length floor mat and repeatedly generates set frequencies and pulses that can restore your body's electric voltage when you lie on the mat for 30 minutes or so daily.[34]

Low-intensity PEMF machines produce less than 1,000 Gauss and are called 'resonance' devices; however high they are turned up you are unlikely to feel much current. High-intensity PEMF machines produce between 1,000–50,000 Gauss and pulse strongly.

IMRS 2000 This machine pulses specific frequencies that restore the body's electric voltage, increasing vitality, improving sleep and stimulating brain function. Regular use improves mental clarity, focus, productivity and mobility, and boosts circulation and immunity, keeping brain ageing at bay.
www.swissbionic.com

Quantron resonance system (QRS) Recommended by NASA, the QRS stimulates the cells – including the brain cells – and boosts the voltage of each one. It reduces inflammation, improves circulation, increases oxygen levels in the blood, boosts cellular energy, and reverses bone density loss.[35]
www.qrs.com

And a few more ideas...

Electromagnetic field (EMF) gauss testing machine

EMFs can play havoc with your brain. In your home or office, the magnetic field should usually be less than 5.0 mG (milligauss) – the electric field less than 20 V/m and the radio frequency (RF) less than 5.0000 mW/m2. Although the fields only matter in the areas that you spend a lot of time, without testing how do you know if you are affected? The Trifield TF2 is the simplest and most comprehensive of the sensors I found. Battery operated, it detects all three types of EMF pollution – AC magnetic, AC electric and radio-frequency microwave – in a single accurate and easy to use unit.
www.trifield.com

Inversion chairs

The health of your brain is connected to how well blood flows around your body. If circulation in or to the brain is restricted, it will impact upon your brain function. Inversion chairs hang you upside down, reversing the effects of gravity, releasing strain on your spinal column and relaxing your muscles. Hanging upside down increases blood flow to your brain and the oxygen in the blood invigorates your brain, boosting your lymphatic system, so enabling it to remove cellular waste more efficiently.

Spirovital oxygen machine

This is a device that uses a patented process, similar to photosynthesis, to create energised, 'activated' air that feeds every cell in your body with oxygen, so boosting your brain function and reducing the effects of ageing, stress, environmental toxins and disease. Unlike standard oxygen therapies, it does not flood the body with oxygen, but instead processes the air that you already breathe to make it more easily usable by the body. Spirovital therapy increases the amount of oxygen the blood releases into the tissues, which increases energy production in the mitochondria as well as the mood boosting happiness hormone, serotonin.

www.spirovital-copdtherapy.com

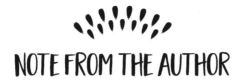

NOTE FROM THE AUTHOR

'Information is not transformation. If you recognise yourself and your patterns, that is information – but what are you going to do to get to the transformation?'

SARA L BRONSON, LIFE COACH

Re-rate your brain energy and function

I hope that the advice and research I've shared with you has taken you on an optimistic, interesting journey and helped you to take action to reboot your own brain. Everyone's journey is different, but now you have worked your way through the questions and exercises, and begun a series of brain-boosting daily practices, how do you feel? My hope is that you'll have a clear sense of mental improvement – increased clarity, energy and improved mood. To check that this is the case, I invite you to repeat the questions you asked yourself at the beginning and flick back to the start of the book to compare your results.

1 On a scale of 1 to 10, where 1 equals exhausted and foggy headed, and 10 is able to think on your feet, feeling energised and well rested, how do you rate your mental energy?

2 On a scale of 1 to 10, where 1 equals very depressed, and 10 is joyful, how do you rate your mood?

3 On a scale of 1 to 10, where 1 equals unable to form clear thoughts, and 10 is able to harness your full brain power to think with clarity and decisiveness, how do you rate your mental clarity?

What's the result?

How have your answers changed from the first time you asked yourself the questions? What do you still need to work on, and how can you incorporate more of the advice, techniques and treatment methods that might support you on the road to further improvement?

The next chapter in my father's story

Hopefully your journey is as positive a one as the road my father and I have travelled. We finally think we have found the major cause of his mental distress – a vast overload of aluminium, mercury and copper in his body. Poor dentistry seems to have been the major culprit, which was a life-changing side-effect that he never signed up for (look back at 'Inside your mouth', Chapter 5). He had a total of 17 implants in his jaw, put in by several different dentists using a variety of metals, many of which had disintegrated over the years. Shocked by the results of his urine and blood tests, my father was determined to have the implants taken out and signed up for extensive surgery: traumatic at any age, but particularly so at 84. The surgeon who removed them said he had rarely seen such toxic, blackened tissue, and that it had extended up his nasal canal and into his brain. The photographs he showed us were like something from a horror movie; little wonder then that my father had problems.

My father recovered from this experience rapidly. Physically he is extremely fit – it was his brain that started failing. The battle that still needs to be won is to remove the unnaturally elevated levels of neuro-toxic copper, mercury and aluminium that remain in his system and still show up in his urine tests. He is currently on a metal detox that will, over the coming months, remove the overload of those metals from his brain. Unfortunately for him, the toxicity of the metals has weakened his kidneys, which means that he can't take advantage of the chelation therapies and pharmaceutical choices that speed up detox. He is having to do it more slowly, yet, in his case, time is of the essence.

A flashing 40Hz light sits on his desk, and his diet is focused. He drinks a bottle of Acilis water a day, and takes a variety of supplements and probiotics at every meal. His mind has, to date, not deteriorated any further and we hope once those metals are finally reduced, that it will improve.

My father's experience underlines yet again how crucial it is for you to take responsibility for your own health. Who knows your body better than yourself? Each of us needs to become our own 'Brain health detective', identify our issues, and then resolve them. I hope this book will show you how.

Let me know how you get on

I would love to hear from you. Any steps you take will undoubtedly move you in the right direction and I cannot stress enough how vital it is to do what you can, and now. Don't hesitate or procrastinate, because any lifestyle or habit change you make now will start benefiting your brain immediately.

The very best of brain rebooting!

With all my good wishes for a brighter, better brain...

Sara x

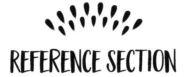

REFERENCE SECTION

CONTENTS

Mind mechanics and brain specialists: how to pick the right expert

I t may be your own brain that concerns you, or you may think someone close to you needs help with theirs – but where or who should you turn to for help? Sometimes a problem is serious; sometimes it isn't. Do you or your friend need psychological assistance or in-depth physical examination and diagnosis? These are important distinctions because the wrong advice could have serious consequences.

So which therapist works best for which particular problem? It is usually best to seek the help of a brain expert for a physical diagnosis and practical physiological help. Find a specialist in the mental and emotional field if you need help to work through past difficulties and present stresses. Often both have a defined role to play in improving your brain health.

The mind 'mechanics'

These are the people you turn to when life feels like it's overwhelming you and your mind feels as if it's no longer your own and you can't control your thoughts and feelings. This includes psychiatrists, psychologists, psychoanalysts, counsellors and therapists, but the list is endless, and when you are struggling to cope it can be hard to make a choice. Wikipedia, for example, currently lists over 155 different types of psychotherapies, so where do you start? Here are some basic guidelines about the main differences – or 'which therapist does what' – that I hope will make your choice as easy as possible.

Psychiatrists

The first big distinction amongst therapists is between psychiatrists and all other experts who offer any kind of mental and emotional advice. Psychiatrists are the heavy hitters; the professionals to guide you when you need serious help. They are trained medical doctors, who then progress to specialising in the vast array of mental health disorders that affect many of us at different times and stages of our lives.

Conditions such as schizophrenia, bipolar, psychosis and acute clinical depression, for example, are serious physical illnesses that cannot be dealt with by counselling or psychotherapy (talking therapies) or be managed by family or friends. Time will not make a difference, and the illness will not just 'pass', but a psychiatrist can make all the difference, and, with proper medical management, symptoms can improve and even normalise.

The precise biochemistry in these conditions is still not properly understood: the brain's neurochemistry is disturbed for one reason or another. The brain chemistry controls behaviour, so symptoms usually include disturbances in emotions, thoughts, moods and behaviour and the only recognised way to treat these illnesses is with medication, and often with intensive and sometimes long-term hospital care or very skilled management in the community. Psychiatrists know what to do and how best to do it, and in the UK they are the only professionals that can prescribe mood and mind-altering (as well as any other) drugs.

Clinical psychologists

Second in line, if you were to categorise the various therapies, would be the clinical psychologists, who are equipped to diagnose and treat emotional and behavioural problems. They can deal with serious mental illness and psychosis. They undergo years of training – a psychology degree, followed by another two or three years at post graduate level. They are skilled at assessing personality and intelligence, and measuring psychological functions in a variety of ways. A clinical psychologist usually has a defined skill, for example, dealing with children, or adolescents, or adults, and may specialise in a specific area – addiction, eating disorders, learning disabilities, education, depression, marital problems, sexual problems, interpersonal conflict management or relationship difficulties in general, for instance.

Make sure the person you go to for help is experienced in your particular issue. Ask around for referrals. Your doctor can offer advice, and if you feel able to talk about your problem to friends you may find they have used a clinical psychologist for exactly the same issue themselves.

Counsellors or psychotherapists (counselling psychologist)

These are the people you can turn to when life seems too difficult to bear – when things seem unmanageable and are causing stress and distress that you can no longer cope with. Counsellors and psychotherapists tend to deal with life traumas and difficulties rather than pathological mental problems. They advise and guide on marital problems, sexual abuse, anxiety, relationship difficulties, eating difficulties, exam stress, bereavement, job anxieties, a difficult child – the problems that many of us deal with through the course of a long life. The terms counsellor or psychotherapist mean pretty much the same thing, and are used interchangeably, though psychotherapists may be more concerned with understanding the past and trying to find ways of resetting it than a counsellor would be.

A counsellor will, on average, have trained for between four and six years, often part time, and during that period they have to look in depth at their own lives and deal with their own issues through personal therapy. London's Tavistock Clinic, Westminster Pastoral Foundation and The British Association of Psychotherapists are all organisations with respected training programmes, and there are many other accredited institutes that regulate the industry. Again, you will need to research the best person for your particular issue.

What is counselling? It comes in many shapes and forms, but generally involves a series of hour-long sessions where you build a safe, trusting relationship with your counsellor, enabling you to talk in depth about your problems and together find coping mechanisms to deal with them. Counsellors don't tell you what to do, but help you work it out for yourself, and help you examine your ways of thinking, and any root causes that may have triggered the problems in the first place.

Psychoanalysts

Psychoanalysis emerged in the 20th century, courtesy of those two greats, Freud and Jung, (see also Chapter 1, About the brain). They fall into two main camps and their followers walk closely in their footsteps.

Sigmund Freud is the grandfather of 'talking therapies' and the originator of the concept of psychoanalysis. He believed that we each have an 'unconscious mind', created by our early life experience, driven primarily by sexual urges, and that these unconscious mental forces are at the root of all adult life issues.

Carl Jung was Freud's protégé, but he came to disagree with his interpretation of the mind, and added an alternative dimension to the concepts of the ego and the individual unconscious, which he called the 'collective unconscious', and declared common to all human beings. Jung believed that each of us arrives at birth with an inherited collection of knowledge and images. He talked of archetypes, universal figures and relationships (mother/child: father/child) – meanings that are the same for all of us, whatever our race or gender – and believed that dream analysis is the way to access the collective unconscious. His ideas link into the modern understandings of a quantum universe, in which there is a consciousness that we ourselves do not create, but that we are beings through which consciousness is experienced – rather like the way gravity is something we experience as a property of our Universe, though we do not create it.

In the first half of the 20th century, these theories came to dominate ways of thinking about human behaviour. Non-medically trained therapists began to be trained as psychoanalysts, developing 'talking cures' for mental difficulties. Freud constructed ideas about the way the mind works that he insisted were true, and for many years they were taken as fact. Patients were required to attend treatment sessions for an hour every day, five days a week and often for years at a time.

Substantial doubt has been thrown in recent time on the accuracy of the way Freud reported his own – now classic – case studies. And there is very little support now for the idea that all disturbances in our psyche are caused by repressed sexual material. Freud saw that the early experiences of life reverberate through the rest of life. But the model he created for how that happens – Id (the primitive part of the mind), ego, superego, repression, dark forces of the unconscious, and so on – bears no systematic relation to how we now know the brain and mind actually work. His model of the mind is only a metaphor, and he himself seems to have been very flawed.[1]

We now know that the mind does not work the way Freud supposed it did, and that his psychoanalytic models have no basis in science. Psychoanalysis lacks any evidence-based research as a treatment for mental issues. It still has its fervent advocates, however, and the training is rigorous and professional, guided by the Institute of Psychoanalysis. Practitioners usually study for a minimum of four years, with three of those years also spent on the couch of a colleague, investigating their own psyche thoroughly.

How to find the right therapist?

The decision to find a therapist can greatly help or hinder your recovery. A good counsellor or therapist will also know when you need medical care, and when medication might help. The best way of finding a therapist is usually through personal recommendation or ask your doctor. Your local Yellow Pages directory will have a list under Psychotherapy or Counselling, or check the Internet. Professional bodies may also have a list of qualified therapists in your area. All of the older, established therapies have a code of ethics, professional associations and training programmes.

It's all about the relationship

In 1940s Chicago, the psychotherapist Carl Rogers developed 'person-centred' psychotherapy. Research showed that the outstanding success of his technique was principally down to the interaction between the therapist and the client, and the therapist's ability to listen to their client with a genuine sense of warmth and empathy. Success was not, as previously thought, based on the therapist's expertise or knowledge, but instead almost entirely on the relationship between the therapist and client. This understanding became central in the wider development of psychotherapy and is at the heart of most of the therapies we recognise as effective today.

Whatever your choice of therapy for mental healing, the relationship you build with your therapist is key to your recovery. So, take your time, and explore your options thoroughly until you find a therapist that works for you, and a therapy you are prepared to commit to.

Ask for a first appointment that will enable you to get a sense of the person you will be working with, and an understanding of whether that therapy will suit your needs. Listen carefully during that session. It's not about what the therapist says they do, their knowledge and experience, or even the organisation they belong to. What makes the difference is the quality of the relationship you sense you can build and the quality of the therapist's ability to empathise and create trust.

And then there are the brain medics

At the same time as you are dealing with the problems of the past and the aspects of life that you struggle with in the present, it is always advisable to reboot your brain biochemistry and address the nutrition and physical choices that can invigorate and balance your brain. And if you have more serious brain issues, then you need correspondingly more serious help.

Naturopathic doctor

The important thing to understand about a naturopathic doctor is that, unlike any conventional medical practitioner, they won't just be looking at your brain. Instead they believe that all parts of your body are linked, and if one area is struggling, there are likely to be clues in other parts as well. They will look back at your long-term health, and they don't believe in suppressing your symptoms, or just treating individual symptoms, but in treating the causes of those symptoms. They examine the roots of what has caused the problem and so then boost your body's natural healing capacity to resolve it itself. Find a consultant who specialises in the brain. They will advise you about diet, supplements and therapies that will improve your situation.

Neurologist

Neuro means 'pertaining to the nervous system', and as the brain is most definitely a part of the nervous system, most brain-related medical words start with the word 'neuro'. Many brain-related illnesses are called neurological diseases. Neurologists are doctors with a specialisation the disorders of the nervous system; they are usually consultants, and often work closely with neurosurgeons.

You may be referred to a neurologist if you have been diagnosed with something that affects your brain and your nerves – multiple sclerosis, Parkinson's, Alzheimer's or Lou Gehrig's diseases, epilepsy, stroke, headaches, seizures or brain infections. They may give you an EEG (electroencephalogram) to establish what is going on in your brain and measure its electrical activity. They can manage your conditions medically, for example, prescribe anti-seizure medications, but are not surgically trained.

Neurosurgeon

If you have been diagnosed with a serious brain illness, such as a brain tumour, stroke or infection of the brain, and have been recommended surgery, you will be referred to a neurosurgeon: a specialist doctor who is trained both to diagnose your symptoms and then to operate to fix them. Find one who has considerable experience.

Neuroradiologist

This is an expert trained to deliver the X-rays, radio waves, ultrasound and magnetic fields used to diagnose and treat brain illnesses. They may scan your brain with a CAT (computed tomography) scan, MRI (magnetic resonance image) or fMRI (functional magnetic resonance image).

Neuropsychologist

Brain injuries can trigger intense emotions ranging from confusion, to anger and despair. A psychologist specifically trained in how brain injuries can affect physical and emotional behaviour, a neuropsychologist can run tests to identify any areas that are damaged and help plan a recovery programme to boost your thinking and memory processes. In some US states neuropsychologists can prescribe medication for depression or to calm someone down – but they can't in the UK. Neuropsychologists can work with you as an individual and also with your family.

Occupational therapist

This is a trained therapist who will help you to manage everyday tasks after an illness or injury, for example. They can help with developing strategies to allow you get on with the things we all take for granted – getting dressed, washing hair, or brushing your teeth. They also work with you to improve your thinking.

Neuro-ophthalmologist

This an eye doctor who specialises in vision problems linked to the brain. Brain injury or illness can leave you with a reduced field of vision, or blurred or sometimes double vision.

Neuro physio and speech therapists

Often when your brain is damaged in some way, different parts of your speech, thinking or movement are affected, depending on which part of the brain has been weakened. Physical or physio therapists will help you to walk and move again, and assist with pain in your back or neck. Speech therapists help with language and cognitive problems – improving organisational skills, reading, writing and understanding – and teach strategies to help memory and planning.

Neurotransmitters and other chemical messengers – the fundamentals of brain function

This is a complicated topic, not least because exactly how all the chemicals circulating in and controlling the body interact with each other is hardly understood at all as yet. The starting point is that there are two main types of chemical messengers in the body: neurotransmitters in the brain and hormones that are released directly into the bloodstream, but some hormones can also cross the blood–brain barrier and enter the brain, and are known as neurohormones. Neurotransmitters, hormones, and neurohormones are the chemical agents that carry messages from one part of the body to the other and control many of our psychological and physical functions. How we sleep, eat, move, and feel, as well as our ability to concentrate and learn, amongst other things, are determined by one or more of them.

Neurotransmitters are produced within the nervous system, and hormones by the endocrine glands – some of which are in or near the brain. Melatonin and cortisol, for example, are hormones produced in the brain, then circulated in the blood, which can affect parts of the body far from their origins. Cortisol has a vast range of functions: it regulates immunity, reduces inflammation, helps control blood pressure, is involved in preparing the body for waking up and going to sleep, and has a massive effect on concentration and attention. It speeds or slows metabolism, regulates blood sugar levels, and boosts the retention of memories. But too much and it becomes the main stress chemical and as such can also destroy brain cells. It is produced by the adrenal glands that sit on top of the kidneys, which is where the fight/flight neurohormone adrenaline comes from too.

What are neurotransmitters?

Nerve cells communicate information to each other using neurotransmitters. They are the brain chemicals, carried by impulses and sent as messages from one set of nerve cells to another via a complex neuron communication network covering the whole of your brain. When an impulse reaches the end of a nerve, it releases a specific neurotransmitter, or chemical, into the gap (called a synapse) between it and the nerve cell on the other side, and passes the message on. The neurotransmitter activates a very specific receptor on the other side of the gap, set up only to receive messages from that particular chemical, so ensuring that each message only reaches its intended recipient. Once it has delivered its message, it is then 'terminated'.

Neurotransmitters either stimulate or calm down any cell they connect with and, as a result, are described as either 'excitatory', or 'inhibitory'. If the neuron connections are not working properly, the receptor that the neurotransmitter attaches to may be faulty, or the neurotransmitter itself is either too strong or not strong enough. That's when brain health issues can arise.

Can you check your neurotransmitter levels?

There is currently no medical way of testing which neurotransmitters in your brain are out of balance. Complementary therapies such as kinesiology (page 213) or Nambudripads's allergy elimination techniques (NAET) can give you an indication as to whether your levels of each are high or low, but otherwise your doctor will advise you according to your symptoms.

Which neurotransmitters affect your brain?

It is not clear how many neurotransmitters there are in total – more than 100 have been identified so far.[1] However, there are six that are particularly important for your brain health and act as the heavy lifters of the system: glutamate, GABA, dopamine, serotonin, acetylcholine and noradrenaline (or norepinephrine).

Glutamate

Glutamate is the neurotransmitter you have – and need – the most of in your brain and central nervous system. It is present at approximately 90 per cent of your brain's synapses. It is your main excitatory neurotransmitter (meaning that it fires up your neurons). It has been shown to boost your brain's capacity to change (its neuroplasticity) and can help your memory and your ability to learn.

If you suffer from headaches, restlessness, anxiety or depression or are super sensitive to pain, then your glutamate levels may be too high. A traumatic event or extreme stress can also raise your glutamate dramatically. Brain overstimulation has been linked to epilepsy, and Alzheimer's, Huntington's and Parkinson's diseases.

Conversely, too little glutamate and your brain will not work as well as it should. Is your memory failing: are you finding it hard to sleep; having difficulty concentrating or remembering; suffering from foggy brain and/or feeling tired all the time? It could be time to top up your glutamate levels. Glutamate is an essential for the memory storage elements of the 'modifiable' synapses in your brain, strengthening or weakening their capacity according to its availability. Low glutamate has also been linked to symptoms of autism, obsessive compulsive disorder (OCD), schizophrenia and depression.

If you have too little glutamate

- **Up your glutamate levels** Buy a supplement in the health store and/or eat more of the foods that contain it naturally, such as meats, dairy products, eggs and high-protein plant foods.

If you have too much glutamate

Inflammation is usually a factor in high-glutamate levels, so try your best to reduce it. (See The second key: Inflammation, action plan, Chapter 2).

- **Take a magnesium supplement** You can take it in pill, capsule, or powder form – the latter goes into your blood stream more rapidly.

- **Other supplements that help** Pyrroloquinolinequinone (PQQ) protects the brain from glutamate toxicity. Coenzyme Q10 lowers glutamate as well as protecting brain cells from free-radical damage.

> ## Did you know...?
> ## A word of warning about MSG
>
> MSG or mono-sodium glutamate is pure glutamate but not something to include on your list of supplements. Found mainly in your Chinese takeaways, the side effects include headaches, sweating and heart palpitations, not to mention the more serious convulsions, diarrhoea, chest pain and mood swings also reported. Asian cooking often includes ginger alongside MSG because, along with Nori and seafood, it protects the brain from over stimulation. Vitamin C protects the receptors that control the release of glutamate in the brain and also protects against the side effects of MSG.

Gamma-aminobutyric acid (GABA)

It is impossible to balance glutamate without looking at your GABA levels too. GABA is as important a neurotransmitter as glutamate and is present in around 90 per cent of the synapses in every part of the brain. Just as glutamate is your main excitatory neurotransmitter, GABA is your major inhibitory neurotransmitter (meaning that it calms nerve impulses down). Together they balance your brain. If you are too wired, stressed or tense, your GABA levels may be low.

If you have too little GABA

- **Take a vitamin B6 supplement** Lack of vitamin B6 (pyridoxine) results in diminished GABA synthesis and a build-up of glutamate. Supplementing may help you relax.

- **Take probiotics** *Lactobacillus brevis* and *Bifidobacterium dentium* have been shown to boost GABA levels. The bacteria in probiotics help improve communication between the gut and brain via the vagus nerve.

- **Add fermented foods to your diet** Sauerkraut, kimchi, kefir and yogurt all increase GABA levels.

- **Take natural plant remedies** Try kava, valerian, lemon balm, chamomile or passionflower; they all enhance GABA levels.

- **Increase your exercise** Exercise raises GABA levels.

- **Sign up for some yoga** Each one hour yoga session has been shown to increase GABA levels by 27 per cent.

If you have too much GABA

This may be a sign that there are problems with your glutamate/GABA balance.

There is an enzyme – Glutamic acid decarboxylase (GAD) – that helps to turn glutamate into GABA, but occasionally it is possible to develop an auto-immune reaction to GAD that means that this process doesn't work properly. If you have coeliac disease, gluten intolerance, Hashimoto's thyroiditis or Type 1 diabetes, this may be an issue. Some people also have a genetic weakness that causes imbalance between glutamate and GABA. Taking mood-altering drugs – both natural and pharmaceutical – can upset it. And if you are stressed and overwired, then endless cups of coffee and tea may not be the best idea for you either, as caffeine increases glutamate activity, while at the same time reducing GABA.

How to balance your glutamate/GABA levels

- **Supplement with taurine** This is an amino acid that binds to GABA receptors in the brain and protects against overly high glutamate levels. Eat seafood (especially shellfish), poultry (especially dark meat), and nori (the seaweed used to wrap sushi) to boost your levels naturally.

- **Increase your exercise** Physical activity corrects glutamate/GABA balance.

- **Supplement with L-theanine** This is a substance that is also structurally similar to both glutamate and GABA that has been shown to stimulate GABA production and slightly lower glutamine levels.

- **Take a vitamin B6 supplement** Vitamin B6 (pyridoxine) is needed to synthesise GABA from glutamate. If you are low in B6 you are likely to have higher glutamate levels.

Dopamine

This neurotransmitter boosts mental focus and memory, along with emotional and sexual arousal, which in turn regulates movement. Dopamine affects mood and is used by the brain's neurons to make movements in response to emotions. Surging levels of dopamine in your brain, triggered by a motivation/pleasure/reward boost, will be, for example, what makes you reach for that second helping of dessert. Low dopamine levels are associated with Parkinson's disease, triggering muscle tremors and problems with moving. Schizophrenia has been linked to high levels of dopamine.

If you have too little dopamine

- **Check vitamin and mineral levels** Take a tyrosine supplement or eat tyrosine-rich foods such as avocados, eggs, fish, chicken, bananas and almonds. Iron, niacin, folate (B9) and B6 are also needed to create dopamine.

- **Sign up for some yoga** Commit to an hour of yoga daily.

- **Spend more time asleep** You need a minimum of seven hours a night.

- **Listen to your favourite music** This is a great way to boost dopamine levels.

- **Incorporate meditation into your day** One hour boosts dopamine production by 64 per cent (see Chapter 9).

- **Go out in the sunshine and take exercise** Sunlight boosts dopamine and improves mood.

If you have too much dopamine

- **Take a vitamin B6 supplement** Up your B6 (pyridoxine) levels and you will reduce your dopamine level.

- **Inhale lemon essential oil** This speeds the turnover of dopamine in the hippocampus.[2]

- **Other supplements/foods that help** Bacopa monnieri balances neurotransmitters; white mulberry, the amino acids 5-HTP (5-hydroxytryptophan) and L-tryptophan found in salmon, dark green leafy vegetables, bananas, nuts, seeds, oats, beans and lentils, tofu, red meat, turkey and eggs, all lower dopamine levels.

Serotonin

Often called the 'calming chemical' because of its ability to modulate moods. Approximately 90 per cent of your serotonin is made in the intestines, with the remainder in the neurons of the central nervous system. In your brain, it helps move messages from one area to another and regulates appetite, sleep patterns, memory and learning, and temperature and behaviour. It also regulates the cardiovascular and endocrine systems, and affects the contraction of muscles. There is a possible link between depression and serotonin too, with lower concentrations of metabolites of serotonin having been found in the cerebrospinal fluid and brain tissue of people suffering from depression.

If you have too little serotonin

- **Increase your exercise levels** This is the fastest and easiest way to raise your serotonin. Vigorous exercise has been shown to keep serotonin levels high for several days afterwards.

- **Add omega-3 fatty acids to your diet** Low levels of omega-3 fatty acids are thought to lower brain levels of serotonin and cause depression.

- **Take L-tryptophan with orange juice at night** Taken just before you go to sleep, the vitamin C converts L-tryptophan into serotonin, which can double serotonin production in your brain.

- **Be cocky about your successes** Very un-British this one, but raise your confidence levels and you increase your serotonin.

If you have too much serotonin

- Few of us suffer from this one – the more serotonin you have in your body, the better your sense of positivity and wellbeing. But your levels can lower by themselves through unhealthy everyday habits like lack of exercise, not getting out in the sunshine, poor diet, or drinking too much coffee (caffeine withdrawal reduces serotonin levels). Change them, and your serotonin levels will rise naturally.

Noradrenaline

This is the 'stress-hormone' neurotransmitter. It prepares your brain (and your body) for action. Stress will trigger the 'fight-or-flight' reaction, which floods noradrenaline (known as norepinephrine in the USA) through your body, increasing your blood pressure and heart rate and boosting the amount of oxygen to your brain – letting you think more quickly and more clearly. Noradrenaline helps with memory and learning, sleep patterns, focus and alertness, and affects circadian rhythm, memory and your perception of pain and reward. Low levels are associated with fibromyalgia, Alzheimer's and Parkinson's diseases and Korsakoff's syndrome, as well as with ADHD, migraines, fatigue and depression. Too much noradrenaline in your system and your anxiety levels will rise, along with your blood pressure, and you may find it harder to sleep at night.

If you have too little noradrenaline

- **Increase your exercise** This raises levels of both noradrenaline and dopamine.

- **Supplement with L-tyrosine or acetyl-L-carnitine** Both increase noradrenaline levels.

- **Increase your noradrenaline-rich foods** Chicken, pure dark chocolate, eggs, meat, bananas, cheese and oatmeal are all good sources.

- **Take supplements** Rhodiola rosea increases levels of noradrenaline, and Asian ginseng increases noradrenaline and dopamine.

- **Try a cold water dip** Extreme cold increases noradrenaline levels by up to 300 per cent in just a few minutes.

- **Go for a sauna** Noradrenaline levels have been found to increase by 100 per cent at 80°C (170°F) and 160 per cent at 100°C (212°F).[3]

If you have too much noradrenaline

- **Supplement with 5-HTP** This amino acid, 5-hydroxytryptophan, reduces norepinephrine.

- **Take melatonin just before going to bed** Melatonin is the sleep hormone and taking it helps reduce the levels of noradrenaline. Noradrenaline makes melatonin and controls its release, so, if you raise your melatonin levels with supplements, your body produces less noradrenaline as its job is done for the time being, but it only works if you take it and then lie down.[4]

Acetylcholine

Found in the brain, and known as the 'memory molecule', acetylcholine helps you stay alert. It is the neurotransmitter that strengthens the vagus nerve, the 'telephone line' which passes messages from your gut to your brain and vice versa. It affects arousal, mood and memory, enhances rapid eye movement (REM) sleep, and boosts brain plasticity. Low levels are associated with Alzheimer's and Parkinson's diseases, myasthenia gravis, and multiple sclerosis. Typically, the brains of patients with Alzheimer's show approximately a 90 per cent loss of acetylcholine.

If you have too little acetylcholine

- **Eat acetylcholine-forming foods** Good sources are eggs and blueberries.

- **Boost your BDNF levels** Regular exercise has been shown to flood the brain with BDNF, a protein that speeds up brain injury recovery and helps to grow new brain cells. Cycling, swimming and running increase BDNF synthesis by 300 per cent.[5] A supplement of 100mg of coffee fruit extract (the red covering over the bean) increases BDNF levels by approximately 140 per cent.[6]

- **Take alpha-GPC** This is a bioavailable form of choline that raises acetylcholine levels.

- **Supplement with citicoline** This is a synthetic substance that mimics a natural substance with neuroprotective benefits and improves memory, focus and attention. Citicoline (CDP-choline), contains choline, a vitamin-like nutrient, a popular ingredient in brain-boosting supplements (nootropics).

- **Supplement with bacopa monnieri** An Ayurvedic herbal remedy, bacopa monnieri (BM) balances neurotransmitters over several months.

- **Try gotu kola** A Chinese, Indonesian and Ayurvedic herbal remedy that in studies has been found to reduce depression and anxiety by 50 per cent and increase mental alertness by 100 per cent.[7]

- **Boost with vitamin B5** The body needs this vitamin to turn choline into acetylcholine.

If you have too much acetylcholine

- **Try kava kava** This is a herbal sedative drink or tea made from the roots of a plant found in the islands of the South Pacific. Research has shown the chemicals in it seem to rectify and balance acetylcholine levels.[8]

- **Cut out foods that contain choline** High-choline foods include fish, meat, poultry, dairy, peanuts and eggs.

Brain-boosting psychobiotics

We know that improving the gut microbiome helps your brain generally (see chapter 8). But you also need to know which psychobiotics (probiotics or prebiotics) will restore your brain function. Plus, how do you know which of the ones you find on the shelf in a health-food store, or On-line, is likely to be worth the money?

There are three checks to make first:

- Does it contain strains that will survive the journey through your stomach's acid?

- Does it need to be kept in the fridge?

- How many strains does the bottle contain – the more there are, the greater the benefit.

Then there are many different strains that help the brain – each one affects in a different way so choose one that addresses your symptoms.

Probiotic	Symptoms that benefit
GG strain	Found to reduce obsessive compulsive disorder (OCD) behaviour in mice and to be as effective as fluoxetine, an anti-depressant often used to treat depression.
J -1 strain of lactobacillus rhamnosus	Has positive effect on the GABA receptors, reducing anxiety, fear and depression in the process. This is one of the few probiotic strains to have been studied in relation to humans as well as rats and mice.
Bifidobacterium longum	Shown in studies to decrease anxiety and depression, as well as impact on paranoia, compulsions and obsessions. Research also shows that this psychobiotic travels via the vagus nerve. Strain 1714 reduces anxiety-linked behaviour; NC 3001 reduces anxiety and normalises behaviour; R0175 also reduces cortisol and improves memory.[1]
Lactobacillus plantarum	Although most of the studies done on this probiotic were carried out on mice, not humans, it does seem to be effective at reducing anxiety. It increases serotonin and dopamine (strain PS128) and was seen to reduce inflammation in depressed mice that had been subjected to early-life stress. Lactobacillus plantarum was found to decrease cortisol, normalise the stress response system (the HPA axis), and decrease depression.[2] A study carried out on people with irritable bowel syndrome (IBS) found that strains CECT7484 and CECT7485 positively affected both their quality of life and their anxiety levels.
Lactobacillus helveticus	This probiotic (strain R0052) reduces cortisol levels, paranoid and obsessive-compulsive thoughts, and anxiety. Strains R0052 and NS8 reduce inflammation in the brain and calm anxiety. Strain ND8 was found to work better than the anti-depressant, citalopram in reducing stress, improving cognitive function and lowering both anxiety and depression levels. It boosted serotonin and lowered cortisol in a rat study.[3] *Lactobacillus helveticus* is found in certain cheeses including Emmental, Cheddar, Parmesan, Romano, provolone and mozzarella.

Lactobacillus reuteri	This bacterium is not found in everyone's gut; some people have it at very low levels, others have none. First discovered in the 1980s, it is one of the best probiotics to take to control inflammation. Timid, withdrawn animals have returned to normal after being treated with it. *Lactobacillus reuteri* reduces stress hormones and alters your GABA receptors. If you suffer from autism, or are socially awkward and anxious, strain 23272 is the one to search out.
	Good for reducing inflammation and boosting antioxidant levels. Take it daily if you suffer from exhaustion, digestive issues or anxiety. It is one of the probiotics found in Yakult.
Lactobacillus casei	In one research study, patients with chronic fatigue syndrome and digestive problems took the Shirota strain of *Lactobacillus casei* daily for two months. By the end of the study, their anxiety symptoms had decreased substantially.

A Japanese study supplemented 20 healthy men over a period of eight weeks with *Lactobacillus casei*. They found that it raised HDL cholesterol levels (the good kind!) and lowered triglycerides much more than the group on a placebo.

Another study gave stressed medical students kefir, a fermented milk drink containing *Lactobacillus casei* strain Shirota, and found that it kept their cortisol levels steady and raised their serotonin levels. It also reduced the side effects of stress – such as stomach cramps and colds.[4] This probiotic is also found in fermented vegetables, dairy products and, oddly, fermented Sicilian green olives. |
| Lactobacillus fermentum | Found in fermented vegetables like kimchi and sauerkraut, it is usually recommended for anxiety, but it reduces inflammation and calms the mind, too. Researchers have found that overuse of antibiotics often triggers acute anxiety, as a consequence of the obliteration of good bacteria in the gut by antibiotics. Strain NS9 will clear up the aftermath and get you back on track again. |
| Bifidobacterium breve | This bacterium is found in human breast milk. The amount in your gut declines as you get older. Research shows that strain 1205 can reduce anxiety-like behaviour, and improve cognitive performance in animals.[5] Unfortunately, I haven't been able to find a psychobiotic supplement that contains it, so up your intake of fermented foods such as sauerkraut and kimchee. |

Galacto-oligosaccharides	Not all psychobiotics are probiotics. Some are 'prebiotics' – non-digestible soluble fibres that stimulate the growth of good gut bacteria. Galacto-oligosaccharides (GOS) is a prebiotic that has been shown to do just that. One study found that GOS significantly decreased the secretion of cortisol, and participants paid more attention to positive information rather than negative information.[6] Other research has demonstrated that people with irritable bowel syndrome (IBS) often have anxiety because of the lack of microbial diversity in their gut. Supplementing with a prebiotic mixture containing GOS significantly reduces their anxiety and improves the quality of their life.[7]
Mycobacterium vaccae	Not all beneficial bacteria enter by mouth. Inhaling *mycobacterium vaccae*, a bacteria found in soil, can improve your mood by stimulating serotonin production. Apparently it activates the same neurons in the brain as the antidepressant Prozac.[8] This may be one of the reasons gardeners feel relaxed and happy when engaging in their favourite pastime. Of course, there's the physical benefit to gardening which raises serotonin – all that digging, mowing and pruning improves oxygen uptake and blood flow.

Did you know...?
Science links gut health with mental health

Two types of gut bacteria have been consistently associated with better mental health - Faecalibacterium and Coprococcus - and both protect against inflammation. The Flemish Gut Flora Project, which studied more than 1,000 people, showed that there was a clear link between the development of depression and having low levels of these two bacteria as well as of a third, Dialister.[9]

Cannabis brain benefits

The fascinating fact about the cannabis plant is that it gives birth to separate male and female plants. Males of the species turn into the down-to-earth hemp plants. The females, however, if left undisturbed by the males, become mind-altering 'marijuana' plants, with an entirely different composition and function altogether. There are two main strains of cannabis – the sativa strains excite and are associated with brain 'highs,' while Indica cannabis creates a state of relaxation. There are hundreds of different combinations of the two, each creating different effects on the body and brain.

The cannabis plant produces very large numbers of different 'cannabinoids', each with a different chemical make-up. The two best known ones are THC and CBD. There are cannabinoid receptors all over your body, in the cell membranes, and particularly in your brain. Research now shows that we probably have more cannabinoid receptors in our bodies than any other receptors and the endocannabinoid system (ECS) may well offer untapped opportunities for healing. The healing effects of the different cannabinoids occur when they activate one of these specific receptors.

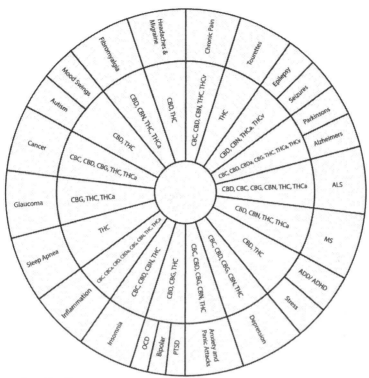

Cannabis Wheel

THC - Tetrahydrocannabinol	**CBD** - Cannabidiol	**CBGa** - Cannabigerol Acid
THCa - Tetrahydrocannabinolic Acid	**CBDa** - Cannabidiolic Acid	**CBC** - Cannabichromenel
THCv - Tetrahydrocannabivarin	**CBG** - Cannabigerol	**CBCa** - Cannabichromenic Acid

Key to the different factors

THC is the one that gets you 'high'. It relaxes you, reduces aggression, and has an effect on pain and inflammation. Used for multiple sclerosis. To reduce its psychoactive effects, balance it with CBD. THC may reverse the ageing process and improve cognitive processes.

THCa is the parent of THC and turns into it when heated. It is considered neuroprotective although its larger molecules don't fit the brain's cannabinoid receptors. Unlike THC, it doesn't make you 'high' and is used for symptoms of glaucoma, fibromyalgia, sleeplessness and pain.

THCv reduces tremors, panic attacks and anxiety levels. Improves brain lesions and motor control problems linked with Alzheimer's.

CBD has no psychoactive component, so no 'highs' from this one either. Good for treating pain, anxiety and inflammation. Used for epilepsy, depression, schizophrenia, ADHD, multiple sclerosis, and motor neurone and Parkinson's diseases.

CBDa is found in raw cannabis flowers and leaves, and is good for inflammation, epilepsy and Alzheimer's and Parkinson's diseases.

CBG promotes apoptosis, or cell death, and protects against nerve cell degeneration in the brain. CBG is the chemical precursor of THC and CBD, effectively their 'parent'. It inhibits GABA uptake and reduces anxiety, depression and paranoia.

CBGa is the cannabis plant's stem cell equivalent and the 'parent' of THCa, CBDa and CBCa.

CBC is a neuron protector, useful for nausea and pain relief.

CBCa is good for inflammation, and is also anti-bacterial

There may, however, be longer term issues...

Although in the short term, the cannabis plant can positively affect a multitude of health issues, do be aware that in the long-term research shows that it lowers the strength of your immune system over time, making it harder to fight off recurrent infections, viruses, bacteria and defend against more serious diseases such as cancer, auto-immune diseases and frailty, which is associated with accelerated ageing.'[1]

Stem cell basics

Stem cells are those that have the ability to change themselves into any other type of cell. So, wherever you have damaged cells, they become whatever is needed to repair the damage, in whichever part of your body is affected.

There are three main types of stem cell, all of which are found in your bone marrow:

Haemopoietic stem cells reboot the immune system.

Mesenchymal stem cells reduce inflammation and turn to muscle and nerve tissue and bone. Mesenchymal stem cells, however, are also found in fat and if that fat is inflamed, when for instance you are overweight, its inflammatory proteins negatively alter their normal function.

Endothelial stem cells strengthen existing blood vessels and make entirely new ones.

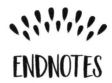

ENDNOTES

Introduction
1. www.telocyte.com
2. Acilis Water www.silicawaters.com

Chapter 1: About the brain
1. Frederick Crews, Freud: the making of an illusion

Chapter 2: Your brain baseline
1. https://www.ncbi.nlm.nih.gov/pubmed/25694817 (accessed 3.5.19)
2. https://www.hindawi.com/journals/jeph/2013/684035/ (accessed 3.5.19)
3. https://waset.org/publications/10000645/environmental-pollution-and-health-risks-of-residents-living-near-ewekoro-cement-factoryewekoro-nigeria (accessed 3.5.19)
4. Horst Eger et al, 'The influence of being physically near to a cell phone transmission mast on the incidence of cancer, Umwelt·Medizin·Gesellschaft 17,4 200
5. https://www.ncbi.nlm.nih.gov/pmc/articles/PMC1480526/
6. Dan Crouse of the University of New Brunswick, a study looking at 1.3 million Canadians in 30 cities over an 11-year period found that living in a 'green' neighbourhood correlated with a 10-year increase in life expectancy.
7. https://www.ncbi.nlm.nih.gov/pmc/articles/PMC4032208/
8. https://www.sciencedirect.com/science/article/pii/S0161813X16302091
9. http://www.rediviva.sav.sk/53i2/59.pdf
10. http://www.abstractsonline.com/Plan/ViewAbstract.aspx?sKey=a9490c38-27f0-4099-8725-3d7eab5e7989&cKey=fcc53b77-f174-4e09-9d22-ccceb76aee81&mKey=54c85d94-6d69-4b09-afaa-502c0e680ca7
11. https://www.ncbi.nlm.nih.gov/pmc/articles/PMC3818819/
12. https://www.telegraph.co.uk/technology/2018/12/10/seven-hours-screen-time-day-changes-structure-childs-brain-scientists/
13. Moskowitz, J, National Toxicology Program report on cancer risk from cell

phone radiation, 7 Sept 2016

14. https://www.ncbi.nlm.nih.gov/pubmed/25478801; https://www.
   mainecoalitiontostopsmartmeters.org/wpcontent/uploads/2013/01/
   Exhibit-10-Smart-Meter-Health-Effects-Report-Survey2.pdf

15. https://www.ncbi.nlm.nih.gov/pmc/articles/PMC2427043/

16. https://engage.gov.bc.ca/app/uploads/sites/391/2018/08/Closer-
   Commutes.pdf

17. https://info.uwe.ac.uk/news/uwenews/news.aspx?id=3713

18. https://journals.plos.org/plosone/article?id=10.1371/journal.pone.0195549

19. https://bjsm.bmj.com/content/49/4/248

20. https://www.ncbi.nlm.nih.gov/pmc/articles/PMC3004979/

21. https://www.ncbi.nlm.nih.gov/pmc/articles/PMC2864873/

22. https://www.imperial.ac.uk/news/183502/london-pollution-cancels-
   positive-health-effects/

23. https://onlinelibrary.wiley.com/doi/full/10.1002/hipo.22427

24. https://www.alzheimers.org.uk/omega-3-and-dementia

25. https://www.ncbi.nlm.nih.gov/pubmed/8327020 – research suggesting
   carnivores have twice the risk of developing dementia than vegetarians,
   perhaps because Alzheimer's correlates with high levels of saturated fat
   in the blood.

26. https://www.ncbi.nlm.nih.gov/pmc/articles/PMC3448747/

27. https://medicalxpress.com/news/2018-11-orange-juice-leafy-greens-
   berries.html

28. A 2-17 Chinese meta-analysis stated that dose-response meta-analysis
   showed that an increment of 100g per day of fruit and vegetable
   consumption was related to an approximately 13 per cent (OR = 0.87, 95
   per cent CI 0.77–0.99) reduction in cognitive impairment and dementia
   risk.

29. https://www.ncbi.nlm.nih.gov/pubmed/12088740 Overview of brain and
   nutrition https://www.ncbi.nlm.nih.gov/pmc/articles/PMC2805706/

30. More than one unit per day has been shown to have a negative
   effect on cognitive function - https://academic.oup.com/jpubhealth/
   article/40/2/304/4793394

31. Sara Davenport, Reboot your health

32. https://www.bda.uk.com/foodfacts/fluid.pdf

33. Blood cholesterol is measured in units called millimoles per litre of blood,
   often shortened to mmol/L. As a general guide, total cholesterol levels
   should be 5mmol/L or less for healthy adults or 4mmol/L for those at
   high risk. LDL cholesterol should be 3mmol/L for healthy adults or 2
   mmol/L for those at high risk. An ideal level of HDL ('bad' cholesterol) is
   above 1mmll/L.

34. https://www.nia.nih.gov/news/loss-vision-associated-loss-cognition,
   worsening vision has been found to correlate with deteriorations in
   cognitive function.

35. Both indicate presence of inflammation

36. https://www.sciencealert.com/side-effects-from-antibiotics-include-
   immune-system-damage-and-fewer-brain-cells-study-shows

37. https://www.ncbi.nlm.nih.gov/pmc/articles/PMC5102822/

38. https://www.bmj.com/content/339/bmj.b2462

39. J Braz, Psychiatry, 2013, Apr-Jun;35(2):193-200

40. https://www.ncbi.nlm.nih.gov/pmc/articles/PMC5579396/

41. Unpredictable stress has been shown to be more psychologically harmful to the brain than stress that can be anticipated.

42. https://www.aarp.org/health/brain-health/info-11-2008/friends-are-good-for-your-brain.html – The same brain changes in Alzheimer's patients with a strong social network are less likely to result in memory impairment when compared to sufferers who don't have support network

43. Occurrence of major stressful experience within the past 12 months correlates with a higher likelihood of depression; multiple stressors magnify the chance. See Holmes-Rahe stress index, Chapter 6.

44. Asa Hakannsson and Goran Molin, 'Gut microbiota and inflammation', Nutrients 2011 June;3(6):637-682

45. Ghasemian M et al, 'Review of anti-inflammatory herbal medicines', AdvPharmacolSci 2016;2016:9130979

46. F Pica et al, 'Serum thymosin a1 levels in patients with chronic inflammatory autoimmune diseases' Clin Exp Immunol. 2016 Oct;186(1):39-45

47. McCollum M, Ma Z, Cohen E, Leon R, Tao R, Wu JY, Maharaj D, Wei J, Post-MPTP, 'Treatment with granulocyte colony stimulating factor improves nigrostriatal function in the mouse model of Parkinson's disease', Molecular Neurobiology 41 (2-3); 410-419, 2010

48. legatus.org/tag/dr-dipnarine-maharaj

49. Science Translational Medicine, 'Health Benefits from Intermittent Fasting', 15 Feb 2017, Vol 9 Issue 377

50. Blackmore, DG et al 2009, 'Exercise increases neural stem cell number in a growth hormone-dependent manner, augmenting the regenerative response in aged mice stem cells', 27:8:2044-52

Chapter 3: Time to detox

1. Needham LL et al, 'Concentrations of environmental chemicals associated with neurodevelopmental effects in the US population', Neurotoxicol. 2005a;26(4):531-545, and Ken Sexton and Dale Hattis, 'Assessing Cumulative Health Risks from Exposure to Environmental Mixtures – Three Fundamental Questions', Environ Health Perspect. 2007 May;115(5); 825-832

2. Hinson JP, 'Effects of endocrine-disrupting chemicals on adrenal function', Best Pract Res ClinEndocrinolMetabl 2006 March;20(1);111-20.

3. https://www.nationalgeographic.com/environment/2018/09/news-air-quality-brain-cognitive-function

4. Medicine & Science, 'Drinking water regularly can have a restorative impact on brain function', Sports & Exercise, June 21, 2018

5. Armstrong LE et al, 'Mild dehyrdration affects mood in healthy young

women', J Nutr.2012 Feb;142(2):382-8

6. Quang Jiang et al, 'Impairment of the glymphatic system after diabetes', Journal of cerebral blood flow & metabolism, July 21, 2016 Vol 37: Issue 4:1326-1337

7. Tanaka M 'Intermittent, moderate-intensity aerobic exercise for only eight weeks reduces artrial stiffness', J Med Ultrason 2013 April, vol 40, Issue 2 119-124

8. S Sundaram, 'Establishing a framework for neuropathological correlates and glymphatic system functioning in Parkinson's disease' Neuroscience and Biobehavioural Reviews, 24 May 2019

9. Hedok Lee et al, 'The effect of body posture on brain glymphatic transport', Journal of Neuroscience, 2015 Aug 5;35(31):11034-11044

Chapter 4: The hidden enemies

1. Readhead B et al, 'Multiscale Analysis of Independent Alzheimer's Cohorts Finds Disruption of Molecular, Genetic, and Clinical Networks by Human Herpesvirus', Neuron Article 1, Vol 99 Issue 1, July 11, 2018. P64-82.

2. Anthony N. van den Pol, 'Viral infection leading to brain dysfunction: more prevalent than appreciated?' Neuron, 2009 October 15;64(1):17-20.

3. Mohammed et al, Neurobiology, Ageing 1992; 13:83-87

4. Mary Holland, Kim Mack Rosenberg and Eileen Iorio, 'The HPV vaccine on trial: Seeking justice for a generation betrayed', Oct 18, 2018 Vaccination, Risk and Failure Reports.

5. CtiradMokráš, Six months administration of BioBran and its effect on high-risk HPV positivity.

6. Neuron, Sam Gandy et al, 'Multiscale analysis of independent Alzheimer's cohorts finds disruption of molecular, genetic and clinical networks by human herpes virus', July 11, 2018, Article 1, Volume 99, Issue 1 pp.64-82

7. Warren-Gash C et al. Association between human herpes virus infections and dementia or mild cognitive impairment: a systematic review protocol. BMJ Open, 2017 Jun 23;7(6):e016522

8. Anna Grahn, 'Varicella-zoster virus (VZV) DNA in serum of patients with VZV central nervous system infections', Journal of infection, 2016; Vol 73; Issue 3:p254-260

9. Lassmann H et al, 'Epstein-Barr virus in the multiple sclerosis brain: a controversial issue' – report on a focused workshop held in the Centre for Brain Research of the Medical University of Vienna, Austria. Brain. 2011 Sep; 134(9): 2772-2786

10. Staras SA et al, 'Seroprevalence of cytomegalovirus infection in the United States, 1988-1994', Nov 2006.Clin. Infect. Dis. 43 (9): 1143-51

11. Elizabeth G Damato, Caitlin W Winnen, 'Cytomegalovirus infection: perinatal implications'. J ObstetGynecol Neonatal Nurs. 2006, 31 (1): 86-92.

12. Brecht, Katharina F et al, 'Postnatal human cytomegalovirus Infection in preterm infants has long-term neuropsychological Sequelae', The Journal of Pediatrics, 166 (4): 834-839

13. Andrew Blauvelt, 'Skin diseases associated with human herpes virus 6, 7, and 8 infection', Journal of Investigative Dermatology Symposium

Proceedings, Volume 6, Issue 3, December 2001, pp. 197–202

14. Josephine M Reynaud and Branka Horvat, 'Human herpes virus 6 and neuroinflammation', ISRN Virology, Volume 2013, Article ID 834890

15. Ben Readhead, 'Multiscale analysis of independent Alzheimer's cohorts finds disruption of molecular, genetic, and clinical networks by human herpes virus', Neuron Vol 99, July 11, 2018, Article 1, Volume 99, Issue 1 pp.64-82

16. Public health England 1 Dec 2016

17. EA Chiocca, CurrOpinMolTher 2008; 10:38-45) Other viruses, such as H1, have been altered too, to provoke an immune attack on cancer cells, Raykov et al, Int J Cancer 2008;122:2880-4

18. Gregory Friedman et al, 'Phase 1 trial safety, tolerability and preliminary efficacy of immune-virotherapy with HSV G207 in children with progressive malignant supratentorial brain tumours', Neuro-oncology, Volume 20, Issue 2, 22 June 2018, pp.i100

19. Annick Desjardins, 'Recurrent glioblastoma treated with recombinant poliovirus', N Engl J Med 2018; July 12. 379:150-161

20. P Billigmann 'Enzyme therapy--an alternative in treatment of herpes zoster. A controlled study of 192 patients', Fortschr Med. 1995 Feb 10;113(4):43-8

21. Wang, L 'The antiviral and antimicrobial activities of liquorice, a widely-used Chinese herb'. Acta Pharm Sin B. 2015 Jul; 5(4): 310–315.

22. Roschek Jr. B et al, 'Elderberry flavonoids bind to and prevent H1N1 infection in vitro', Phytochemistry. 2009;70(10):1255-61

23. Stefanie Johnson et al, 'Risky Business: linking toxoplasma gondii infection and entrepreneurship behaviours across individuals and countries', Proceedings of the Royal Society, 25 July 2018, Vol 285, Issue 1883

24. Lengerich EJ, et al, 'Severe giardiasis in the United States', Clin Infect Dis 1994; 18: 760-763

25. Berkmann DS et al, 'Effects of stunting, diarrhoeal disease, and parasitic infection during infancy on cognition in late childhood: a follow-up study', Lancet 2002; 359: 564-571

26. Jones-Brando L et al, 'In vitro inhibition of toxoplasma gondii by four new derivatives of artemisinin', Antimicrob Agents Chemother 2006. 50:4206-4208

27. Pillai S et al, 'Anti-parasitic activity of myristica fragrans houtt essential oil against toxoplasma gondii parasite', APCBEE Procedure, 2012, vol 2; pp.92-96

28. Jaiswal P, 'Biological effects of myristica fragrans', Annu Rev Biomed Sci 2009;11:21-29

29. Krivogorsky B et al, 'Structure-activity studies of some berberine analogs as inhibitors of toxoplasma gondii', Bioorg Med Chem Lett, 2012 Apr 15;22(8):2980-2

30. 31. WHO guidelines on indoor air quality: dampness and mould

32. Mudarri and Fisk, 2007

33. Eileen Scully et al, 'Fungal brain infections', Current opinion Neurology 2008:21:347-352

34. https://www.sciencenews.org/article/mold-may-mean-bad-news-brain

35. B Robert Crago and Michael R Gray et al, 'Psychological, neuropsychological and electrocortical effects of mixed mold exposure', Arch Environ Health, 2003 Aug;58(8);452-63. Also Michael R Gray, 'Molds, mycotoxins and public health – eckleylaw.com.

36. CF Harding et al, 'Mold inhalation, brain inflammation and behavioural dysfunction' Nov 15, 2104 Presentation Neuroscience 2014: http://www.abstractsonline.com/Plan/ViewAbstract.aspx?sKey=a9490c38-27f0-4099-8725-3d7eab5e7989&cKey=fcc53b77-f174-4e09-9d22-ccceb76aee81&mKey=54c85d94-6d69-4b09-afaa-502c0e680ca7. Shenassa ED et al, 'Dampness and mold in the home and depression:an examination of mold-related illness and perceived control of one's home as possible depression pathways', Am J. Public Health, 2007;11:65-74. Crago BR et al, 'Psychological, neuropsychological and electro-corticol effects of mixed mold exposure', Arch Environ Health 2003 Aug; 58(8);452-63 (hypoactivation of the frontal lobe). Baldo JV et al, 'Neuropsychological performance of patients following mold exposure', Appl Neuropsychol 2002. 9(4):193-202 (visuospatial learning, visuospatial memory, verbal learning and psychomotor speed all impaired. Also depression).

37. Stephen A Klotz et al, 'Fungal and Parasitic infections of the Eye', Clinical microbiology reviews, American Society for Microbiology

38. As footnote 35 above

39. Alsonso R et al, 'Cerebrospinal fluid from Alzheimer's disease patients contains fungal proteins and DNA', J Alzheimer's Dis. 2015, 47, 873-876

40. Dr David B Corry, 'Microglia and amyloid precursor protein coordinate control of transient Candida cerbritis with memory deficits', Nature Communications 10, 2019, article number:58

41. Journal ApplNutr 1995;47:96-102

42. 'Is 5G dangerous?', BCS, 25 Feb 2019, and irseco.com/European-union-5G-appeal-scientists-warn of-potential-serious-health-effects of-5G

43. A B Miller, 'Cancer epidemiology update, following the 2011 IARC evaluation of radiofrequency electromagnetic fields', Monograph 102, Environ Res, 2018 Nov;167:673-683

44. Khurana V et al Cell phones and brain tumours: a review including the long-term epidemiologic data'Surgical Neurology' Vol 72 Issue 3 Sept 2009 p 205-214

45. Kaplan S et al 'Electromagnetic field and brain development Journal of Chemical neuroanatomy Vol 75, Part B, September 2016, pp.52–61

46. S A Meo, 'Mobile phone base station tower settings adjacent to school buildings: Impact on students cognitive health', American Journal of Men's Health, Vol 13, Issue 1, Jan 1 2019

47. Lai and Levitt 2010, 'Biological effects from exposure to electromagnetic radiation emitted by cell tower base stations and other antenna arrays', Environmental Reviews 18(1):369-395 Feb 2010

Chapter 5: The skull is not a sealed box

1. Mornstad, Teivens, Wanman, 'Health status and attitudes to amalgam.

A questionnaire to members of the Dental Patient Organisation Tandlakartidningen 86, 1994, 196-204

2. British Society for Ecological Medicine 'Systemic effects of metal exposure in clinical practice: protecting patients and optimizing outcomes', 16 Nov 2018

3. Stajskal V et al, 'The role of metals in autoimmunity and the link to neuroendocrinology' Neuroendocrinology Letters 1999;20:353-5

4. https://www.ncbi.nlm.nih.gov/pmc/articles/PMC4642684/

5. As footnote 2 above plus, Bjorklund G et al, 'Metals and Parkinson's disease: mechanisms and biochemical processes', Curr Med Chem, 2017. Stjskal V, 'Allergy and autoimmunity caused by metals: a unifying concept', Vaccines and Autoimmunity: John Wiley & Sons; 2015. Stjskal V et al, ' The role of metals in autoimmunity and the link to neuroendocrinology', Neuroendocrinology letters, 1999;20:353-3

6. KarthikSivaraman et al, 'Is zirconia a viable alternative to titanium for oral implant? A critical review', Japan Prosthodontic Society, 2017

7. Hallab N et al, Elizabeth Valentine-Thon et al, 'LTT-Melisa is clinically relevant for detecting and monitoring metal sensitivity', J. Bone Joint Surg 2001;3(83A):428.

8. Anu Sharma, 'Neuroplasticity in deafness: evidence from studies of patients with cochlear implants, University of Colorado

9. Isabelle Mosnier et al, 'Improvement of cognitive function after cochlear implantation in elderly patients', JAMA Otolaryngology-Head & Neck surgery, 12 March 2015

10. Lelic D, Niazi IK, Holt K, Jochumsen M, Dremstrup K, Yielder P, Murphy B, Drewes AM, and Haavik H, 'Manipulation of dysfunctional spinal joints affects sensorimotor integration in the pre-frontal cortex: A brain source localisation study,' Mar 7, 2016 Neural Plasticity. Kent C, Neuroimmunology and chiropractic, The Chiropractic Journal, October 1995. Tuchin PJ, 'The effects of spinal manipulaton on the Immune system' ACA Journal of Chiropractic and Osteopathy 2: 1998 pp 86–92

11. Brenna P et al, 'Enhanced phagocytic cell respiratory bursted induce by spinal manipulation: potential role of substance P', J Manip, Physiolog Ther 1991; (14)7:399-400

12. The Sid E Williams Research Centre of Life Chiropractic University adjusted a group of HIV positive patients over a 6-month period. They found that patients that were adjusted had an increase of 48 per cent in the CD4 cells (an important immune system marker). The control group in contrast had a 7.96 per cent decrease in CD4 numbers.

13. Selano JL et al, 'The effects of specific upper cervical alignments on the CD4 counts of HIV-positive patients', The Chiro Research Journal;3(1);1994

14. Tony St Leger, 'Bacteria live on our eyeballs – and understanding their role could help treat common eye diseases', The Conversation, 21 June 2019

15. Romulus P, 'Glaucoma and disability: which tasks are affected and at what stage of disease?' Curr Opinion Ophthalmol (Internet) 2009;20

16. Exp Eye Res 2012;101:9-15, Macushield.com.

17. Int J Ophthalmol, 2016;9:145-52

18. J Neuro Sci Res, 2018, 96; 731-43

19. Farzad Salehpour et al, 'Brain Photobiomodulation therapy: A narrative review', Mol Neurobiol. 2018, Aug:55(8):6601-6636

20. Artin Arshamian et al, 'Respiration modulates olfactory memory consolidation in humans', Journal of Neuroscience 28 November 2018, 38 (48) 10286-10294; DOI: https://doi.org/10.1523/JNEUROSCI.3360-17.2018. Bakris G et al, 'Atlas vertebra realignment and achievement of arterial pressure goal in hypertensive patients: a pilot study', Journal of Human Hypertension 2007, 21, 347-352

21. Northumbria University, Newcastle, 'Herbs that can boost your mood and memory', 29 April 2016, Dept of Psychology. Presented at the annual British Psychological Society Conference, Nottingham, 26–28 April 2016

22. https://www.ncbi.nlm.nih.gov/pubmed/22612017

23. Sayowan W et al, 'The effects of jasmine oil inhalation on brain wave activities and emotions', Journal of Health Research 27 (2) 73-77, March–April 2013

24. Yuri P Danilov et al, 'Electrical tongue stimulation normalises activity within the motion-sensitive brain network in balance-impaired subjects as revealed by group independent component analysis' Brain Connect. 2011 Sep; 1(3): 255-265

Chapter 6: Emotions and their effect on the brain

1. McManus S, Meltzer H, Brugha T S, Bebbington P E, and Jenkins R, Adult psychiatric morbidity in England, 2007: results of a household survey. The NHS Information Centre for health and social care. Pub. 2009

2. Stacey Vornbrock, 'Role of the conscious and subconscious Minds – www.breakthroughperformance.net

3. https://www.ncbi.nlm.nih.gov/pmc/articles/PMC2694920/

4. As note 3, above

5. https://www.ncbi nlm.nih.gov/pmc/articles/PMC4461089/

6. https://www.ncbi.nlm.nih.gov/pubmed/18494537

7. https://www.health.harvard.edu/blog/sad-depression-affects-ability-think-201605069551

8. https://doi.org/10.1192/bjp.bp.112.118307

9. https://www.ncbi.nlm.nih.gov/pmc/articles/PMC5327822/

10. https://www.ncbi.nlm.nih.gov/pmc/articles/PMC3302010/

11. Joergensen el al, 2011

12. Holmes-Rahe Stress Inventory; American Institute of Stress

13. P Brown and T Dzendrowskyj, 'Sorting Out an Emotional Muddle', Developing Leaders, Issue 29. Spring 2018

13. Jina Park et al, 'Meaning in life and adjustment to daily stressors', Journal of Positive Psychology, vol 12 2017 – Issue 4

14. Catherine Nakonetschny, 'Cultivating a sense of purpose in people with dementia' Social Work Today. Leider R et al, 'The Power of Purpose: Find meaning, live longer, better', pub. Barrett Koehler Publishers, 2015

15. https://time.com/5511729/monk-mindfulness-art-of-dying/

16. Fredrickson 2013

Chapter 7 Action! What to eat and how to move

1. Pauline H Croll et al, 'Better diet quality relates to larger brain tissue volumes: The Rotterdam Study', Neurology May 16 2018

2. https://academic.oup.com/ajcn/article/90/3/680/4597089

3. https://www.thenation.com/article/warning-signs-how-pesticides-harm-young-brain/

4. Environmental Working Groups annual analysis of US Dept of Agriculture 'Dirty Dozen' list Feb 2019

5. UK Soil Association survey, Organic farming, food quality and human health: A review of the evidence

6. https://www.independent.co.uk/life-style/health-and-families/health-news/organic-pesticide-linked-with-parkinsons-disease-622080.html

7. 'Best and worst foods for pesticide residues in the UK, Aug 31, 2017, UK food studies 2011-15, issuu.com

8. Shukitt-Hale B, Lau F, Joseph J, 'Berry fruit supplementation and the ageing brain', J. Agric. Food Chem., 2008, 56 (3), pp 636–641DOI: 10.1021/jf072505f

9. https://www.ncbi.nlm.nih.gov/pubmed/26254971

10. Khushbu K Modi et al, 'Cinnamon converts poor learning mice to good learners: Implications for memory improvement', Journal of Neuroimmune Pharmacology, 2016

11. https://www.ncbi.nlm.nih.gov/pubmed/10400551

12. https://www.ncbi.nlm.nih.gov/pubmed/24150106

13. Bauer I, Hughes M, Rowsell R, Cockerell R, Pipingas A, Crewther S, and Crewther D 'Omega-3 supplementation improves cognition and modifies brain activation in young adults', 2014, Hum. PsychopharmacolClinExp, 29: 133-144. doi:10.1002/hup.2379

14. White DJ, de Klerk S, Woods W, Gondalia S, Noonan C, Scholey AB, 'Anti-stress, behavioural and magnetoencephalography effects of an L-Theanine-Based Nutrient Drink: A randomised, double-blind, placebo-controlled, crossover trial', Nutrients 2016;8.

15. Ale-Agha N, Goy C, Jakobs P, Spyridopoulos I, Gonnissen S, Dyballa-Rukes N, et al, 'CDKN1B/p27 is localised in mitochondria and improves respiration-dependent processes in the cardiovascular system—new mode of action for caffeine. 2018, PLoSBiol 16(6): e2004408. https://doi.org/10.1371/journal.pbio.2004408

16. Astrid Nehlig Br J, 'The neuroprotective effects of cocoa flavanol and its influence on cognitive performance', ClinPharmacol. 2013 Mar; 75(3): 716-727

17. Sabelli H et al, 'Sustained antidepressant effect of PEA replacement', J Neuropsychiatry ClinNeurosci. 1996 Spring:8(2); 168-71

18. Enkephalin: Kelley AE1, Will MJ, Steininger TL, Zhang M, Haber SN. 'Restricted daily consumption of a highly palatable food (chocolate ensure(R)) alters striatal enkephalin gene expression.' Eur J Neurosci. 2003 Nov;18(9):2592-8.

19. https://www.ncbi.nlm.nih.gov/pubmed/20838622

20. http://www.jneurosci.org/content/34/46/15139.abstract

21. https://www.ncbi.nlm.nih.gov/pubmed/20590847

22. https://thrivous.com/blogs/views/dr-parker-on-brain-and-body-benefits-from-alcar-and-alpha-lipoic-acid

23. https://www.ncbi.nlm.nih.gov/pubmed/18065594 and https://www.ncbi.nlm.nih.gov/pubmed/17658628

24. https://www.ncbi.nlm.nih.gov/pubmed/28992629

25. https://www.sciencedirect.com/science/article/pii/S0939475318301248

26. https://www.ncbi.nlm.nih.gov/pubmed/29704637

27. https://www.ncbi.nlm.nih.gov/pmc/articles/PMC3501277/

28. https://news.cornell.edu/stories/2008/02/scientists-close-taurines-activity-brain

29. https://www.nature.com/articles/1395862

30. https://www.ncbi.nlm.nih.gov/pmc/articles/PMC3746283/#B66

31. https://www.ncbi.nlm.nih.gov/pmc/articles/PMC3933742 (accessed 4.5.19)

32. https://www.ncbi.nlm.nih.gov/pubmed/17367269 (accessed 4.5.19)

33. https://www.sciencedirect.com/science/article/pii/S0301008214000124 (accessed 4.5.19)

34. https://openheart.bmj.com/content/5/2/e000784

35. Russell T Matthews et al, 'Coenzyme Q10 administration increases brain mitochondrial concentrations and exerts neuroprotective effects', Proc Natl AcadSci USA, 21 July 1998;95(15):8892-8897

36. https://www.consumerlab.com/answers/how-does-turmeric-spice-differ-from-turmeric-curcumin-supplements/tumeric_spice_vs_supplements (accessed 4.5.19)

37. https://www.sciencedirect.com/science/article/pii/S1064748117305110?via per cent3Dihub

38. http://www.ipsen.com/en/encouraging-results-guidage-large-scale-european-trial-conducted-prevention-alzheimer-s-dementia.

39. Duffy S et al, ' Glutathione relates to neuropsychological functioning in mild cognitive impairment', Alzheimer's and Dementia: The Journal of the Alzheimer's Assoc;10:67-75 2014

40. Wattanathorn J et al, 'Positive modulation of cognition and mod in the health elderly volunteer following the administration of centella asiaica', J Ethnopharmacol, 5 Mar 2008;116(2):325-32

41. https://www.ncbi.nlm.nih.gov/pmc/articles/PMC4137276

42. https://www.ncbi.nlm.nih.gov/pubmed/24086396

43. https://journals.sagepub.com/doi/10.1177/107385840000600607 (accessed 4.5.19)

44. https://www.ncbi.nlm.nih.gov/pubmed/22326943

45. https://www.ncbi.nlm.nih.gov/pmc/articles/PMC6158605

46. https://www.ncbi.nlm.nih.gov/pubmed/24077207

47. https://www.ncbi.nlm.nih.gov/pmc/articles/PMC4404917

48. https://www.ncbi.nlm.nih.gov/pubmed/25933483

49. https://www.ncbi.nlm.nih.gov/pubmed/17713111

50. https://www.ncbi.nlm.nih.gov/pmc/articles/PMC4772032/

51. https://www.ncbi.nlm.nih.gov/pmc/articles/PMC2649700 (accessed 4.5.19)

52. https://www.ncbi.nlm.nih.gov/pmc/articles/PMC4276978 (accessed 4.5.19)

53. https://www.ncbi.nlm.nih.gov/pubmed/10400551 (accessed 4.5.19)

54. Heike A, Bischoff-Ferrari M, et al, 'A pooled analysis of vitamin D dose requirements for fracture prevention', New Engl Med, 2012; 367; 40-9

55. Le Blanc E et al, 'Associations between 25-Hyroxyvitamin D and weight gain in elderly women', Journal of Women's Health, 2012; 20 (10): 1066-73

56. https://www.ncbi.nlm.nih.gov/pubmed/22536767 (accessed 4.5.19)

57. https://www.ncbi.nlm.nih.gov/pubmed/7082716

58. https://www.alzheimers.org.uk/info/20010/risk_factors_and_prevention/136/physical_exercise

59. https://press.rsna.org/timssnet/media/pressreleases/14_pr_target.cfm?ID=1921

60. 16a Matthew M Robinson et al, ' Enhanced protein translation underlies improved metabolic and physical adaptation to different exercise training modes in young and old humans', Cell Metabolism, March 07 2017 Vol 25 Issue 3 pp.581-592

61. Colcombe et al, 2003

62. Thomas AG, Dennis A, Bandettini PA, Johansen-Berg H, 'The effects of aerobic activity on brain structure', Front Psychol. 2012;3:86. Published 2012 Mar 23. doi:10.3389/fpsyg.2012.00086

63. https://www.ncbi.nlm.nih.gov/pmc/articles/PMC4640257/

64. Robinson M, Sreekuman Nair et al 'Enhanced protein translation underlies improved metabolic and physical adaptations to different exercise training modes in young and old humans', Cell Metabolism, 25, 581-592 March 7 2017

65. https://www.physiology.org/doi/full/10.1152/japplphysiol.00126.2015

66. Hamer, M et al, 'Association of body mass index and waist-to-hip ratio with brain structure', American Academy of Neurology Jan 9, 2019

67. Davis JC, et al, 'Sustained cognitive and economic benefits of resistance training among community-dwelling senior women: a 1-year follow-up study of the Brain Power study. 2010, Archives of Internal Medicine, 170(22), 2036-2038. https://jamanetwork.com/journals/jamainternalmedicine/fullarticle/776438

68. https://www.uea.ac.uk/about/-/it-s-official-spending-time-outside-is-good-for-you

69. Erickson KI et al, 'Physical activity predicts gray matter volume in late adulthood: The Cardiovascular health study. Neurology, 2010, 75(16), 1415-1422.

70. https://www.ncbi.nlm.nih.gov/pmc/articles/PMC4428135/

71. https://www.ncbi.nlm.nih.gov/pmc/articles/PMC3289222/

72. https://www.pnas.org/content/115/41/10487

Chapter 8: The gut brain, the heart brain and hormones

1. J Psychiatr Res, 2015 Apr;63:1-9. doi: 10.1016/j.jpsychires.2015.02.021. Epub 2015 Mar 3.

2. Amar Sarkal et al, 'Psychobiotics and the manipulation of bacteria-gut-brain signals', Trends Neurosci. 2016 Nov; 39(11): 763-781.

3. https://www.ncbi.nlm.nih.gov/pmc/articles/PMC4977816/#b5-cpn-14-231

4. https://www.sciencedaily.com/releases/2018/04/180414171634.htm

5. Wall R, Cryan JF, Ross RP, Fitzgerald GF, Dinan TG, and Stanton C, 'Bacterial neuroactive compounds produced by psychobiotics', AdvExp Med Biol. 2014;817:221-39. doi: 10.1007/978-1-4939-0897-4_10

6. NobuyukiSudo, et al, 'Postnatal microbial colonisation programs the hypothalamic–pituitary–adrenal system for stress response in mice', J Physiol. 2004 Jul 1; 558(Pt 1): 263–275

7. TG Dinan et al, J.Psych. res 2015/www.ncbi.nlm.nih.gov/pubmed/25772005

8. https://doi.org/10.1016/j.clnu.2018.04.010

9. Wilson et al, 'Cytokines and cognition – the case for a head to toe inflammatory paradigm', JAGs 50;2041-2056,2002

10. Shen et al, 'Bioenergetic state regulates innate inflammatory responses', Nature 2017;8(624)

11. https://www.ncbi.nlm.nih.gov/pmc/articles/PMC3547419

12. Queensland University of Technology, 'Decisions under pressure: It's all in the heartbeat', Science Daily, 17 July 2008.

13. Thacker EL et al, 'Atrial fibrillation and cognitive decline: a longitudinal cohort study', Neurology, July 9 2013 :81(2);119-25

14. R McCraty, 'New frontiers in heart rate variability and social coherence research: techniques, technologies and implications for improving group dynamics and outcomes', Frontiers in Public Health, 12 October 2017

15. Delarue J et al, 'Fish oil prevents the adrenal activation elicited by mental stress in healthy men', Diabetes Metab. 2003 June:29(3):289-95

16. Spiegel K et al, 'Impact of sleep debt on metabolic and endocrine function', Lancet 1999, Oct 23;354((9188):1435-9

Chapter 9: Daily practices

1. Roeser R et al, 'Mindfulness training and reductions in teacher stress and burnout: Results from two randomised, waitlist-control field trials', Journal of Educational Psychology, Vol 105(3), Aug 2013, 787-804

2. Chiesa, Calati and Serretti, 2011

3. S W Lazar, 'Meditation experience is associated with increased cortical thickness', Neuro Report, 2005 Nov 28;16(17):1893-1897

4. https://www.ncbi.nlm.nih.gov/pubmed/23541163

5. https://www.thelancet.com/journals/lancet/article/PIIS0140-6736(14)62222-4/fulltext

6. Carson et al, 'Loving kindness meditation for chronic low back pain:

Results from a pilot trial', Journal of Holistic Nursing, Sept 1 2005

7. Sandra Manninen et al, 'Social laughter triggers endogenous opioid release in humans', Journal of Neuroscience, 2017; 0688-16

8. S Anderson et al, 'Reversal of age-related neural timing delays with training', Neuroscience 2013 Mar 12;110(11):4357-4362

9. R L Smith-Ray 'Impact of cognitive training on balance and gait in older adults', Journal of Gerontology Series B 2015 May;70(3):357-66

10. https://mic.com/articles/110662/science-shows-something-surprising-about-people-who-still-journal#.9iQgPSezv

11. Robert A Emmons 'Gratitude, Subjective Well-being and the Brain', APA psychnet, 2008

12. Robert A Emmons and Michael McCullough, 'Counting blessings versus burdens: an experimental investigation of gratitude and subjective well-being in daily life' Journal of Personality and Social Psychology, 2003, Vol 84 No2, 377-389

13. Adam P Spira et al, 'Impact of Sleep on the Risk of Cognitive Decline and Dementia', Current Opinion in psychiatry, Nov 2014 ;27(6): 474–483

14. https://www.nih.gov/news-events/nih-research-matters/sleep-deprivation-increases-alzheimers-protein

15. https://www.sciencedaily.com/releases/2014/06/140605141849.htm

16. Nedergaard et al 'Sleep drives metabolite clearance from the Adult Brain' Science 2013 Oct 18;342(6156)

17. https://www.ncbi.nlm.nih.gov/pubmed/26211735

Chapter 10: Complementary therapies that boost the brain

1. Gerhardt Litscher, 'Violet Laser acupuncture – Part 1: effects on brain circulation', Journal of Acupuncture and Meridian Studies Volume 3 Issue 4, December 2010, pp.255–259

2. Gay CW et al, 'Immediate changes after manual therapy in resting state functional connectivity as measured by fMRI in participants with induced low back pain', Journal of Manipulative and Physiological Therapeutics. 37(9). 2014.

3. Richard Barwell et al, 'The effect of the chiropractic adjustment on the brain wave pattern as measured by QEEG: A four case study summarizing an additional 100 (approximately) cases over a three year period.' (D.C.) http://www.worldchiropracticalliance.org/tcj/2008/jun/n.htm

4. Daniel Cherkin et al, 'Effect of mindfulness-based stress reduction vs cognitive behavioural therapy or usual care on back pain and functional limitations in adults with chronic low back pain', JAMA 2016 March 22/29

5. Patrícia Ribeiro Porto et al, 'Does cognitive behavioural therapy change the brain? A systematic review of neuroimaging in anxiety disorders', Journal of Neuropsychiatry, April 1 2009 publ online.

6. Guillermo A Matarán-Peñarrocha-Penarrocha et al, 'Influence of craniosacral therapy on anxiety, depression and quality of life in patients with fibromyalgia' Evid Based Complement Alternat Med. 2011. 178769. Heidemarie Haller, MSc, 'Craniosacral therapy for the treatment of chronic neck pain. A randomised sham-controlled trial', Clin J Pain 2016;32:441–

449)

7. Paul Swingle et al, 'Neurophysiological indicators of EFT treatment of post-traumatic stress', Subtle energies and energy medicine Vol 15; p76). Dawson Church, 'Clinical EFT as an evidence-based practice for the treatment of psychological and physiological conditions'. Psychology 2013. Vol.4, No. Anxiety

8. Gary Craig, 'Emotional freedom techniques (EFT) For traumatic brain injury', Holistic healing publications May 2009; Vol 9, No 2

9. Bach et al, 2016

10. Sander Nieuwenhuis et al, 'Bilateral saccadic eye movements and tactile stimulation, but not auditory stimulation, enhance memory retrieval', 2012

11. Helen J Crawford, 'Brain dynamics and hypnosis: Attentional and disattentional processes', International Journal of Clinical and Experimental Hypnosis. Volume 42, 1994 – Issue 3, pp.204-232

12. Akaike A, 'Protective effects of a vitamin B12 analog, mehtylcobalamin, against glutamate cytotoxicity in cultured corticol neurons'. Eur J PHarmacol. 1993 Se 7;241(1(:1-6

13. Schmitt, W, 'Correlation of Appplied Kinesiology Muscle Testing Findings with Serum Immunogobulin Levels for Food Allergies' International Journal of Neuroscience, 1998 vol 96: Issue 3-4 p 237-244

14. Riggs, S, 'My brain needs oxygen – what can I do?', NACD Foundation, 2012 Vol 25 No 5

Chapter 11: Machines that stimulate your brain

1. H Geeseink and D Meijer, 'Quantum wave information of life revealed: An algorithm for electromagnetic frequencies that create stability of biological order, with implications for brain function and consciousness', NeuroQuantology, March 2016, Vol 14, Issue 1, pp.106–125

2. Concussion Alliance 'Light Therapy (Photobiomodulation)', concussionalliance.org

3. M Schweitzer et al, 'Healing spaces: Elements of environmental design that make an impact on health', JACM, Vol 10, No 1, 22, Oct 2004

4. T Cesarz et al, 'The effects of blue and red light on physiological responses post-exercise', University of Wisconsin-Madison, 2015

5. Elixa.com, 'Healing with single frequency LED light'

6. www.sota.com, LightWorks

7. Tian F, Hase SN, Gonzalez-Lima F, et al, 'Transcranial laser stimulation improves human cerebral oxygenation', Lasers Surg Med. 2016 Apr;48(4):343-9. Hamblin MR, 'Shining light on the head: Photobiomodulation for brain disorders', BBA Clin. 2016 Dec; 6: 113-124.

8. Barrett DW, Gonzalez-Lima F, 'Transcranial infrared laser stimulation produces beneficial cognitive and emotional effects in humans', Neuroscience 230 (2013) 13-23

9. F. Gonzalez-Lima and Douglas W Barrett, 'Augmentation of cognitive brain functions with transcranial lasers', Front. Syst. Neurosci., 14 March 2014

10. www.ncbi.nlm.nih.gov/pmc/articles/PMC5568598/

11. 'Navigation and spatial memory: New brain region identified to be involved', Science Daily, 16 August 2017

12. Kang et al, 2009, 'Slow wave sleep disruptions increases cerebrospinal fluid amyloid B levels', Bran 2017, Aug:140(8):2014-2111

13. Gruzelier, 'A theory of alpha/theta neurofeedback, creative performance enhancement, long distance functional connectivity and psychological integration', Cogn Process 2009 Feb;10 Suppl 1

14. Ahmed and Wieraszko, 'The mechanism of magnetic field-induced increase of excitability in hippocampal neurons', Brain Res, 2008 July 24;1221:30-40

15. Cosic, Cosic and Lazar, 'Is it possible to predict electromagnetic resonance in proteins, DNA and RNA?' EPJ Nonlinear Biomedical Physics, Dec 2015, 3:5

16. Sisken, Midkiff, Tweheus & Markhov, 'Nanomedicine opens the way for nerve cell regeneration', Science News May 21, 2007, Elsevier Health Sciences

17. Lee et al 2006, 'Efficacy of pulsed electromagnetic therapy for chronic lower back pain: A randomised, double-blind, placebo-controlled study', Journal of International Medical Research. 34(2), 160

18. Sakai, Suzuki, Nakamura, et al, 'Effects of pulsing electromagnetic fields on cultured cartilage cells', Int Orthop. 1991;15(4):341-6

19. Tekutskaya, Barishev and Ilchenko, 'The effect of a low frequency electromagnetic field on DNA molecules in aqueous solutions', semanticsscholar.org. 2015,

20. Yu et al, 'Activation of the anterior prefrontal cortex and serotonergic system is associated with improvements in mood ad EEG changes induced by Zen meditation practice in novices'. Int. Journal of psychophysiology Vol 80 Issue 2, May 2011

21. Otis Smart et al, 'Multimodal approaches to define network oscillations in depression', published online Biological Psychiatry, Jan 27, 2015

22. G Buzsaki 'Hippocampal sharp wave-ripple: A cognitive biomarker for episodic memory and planning', Hippocampus 2015, Oct; 25(10):1073-1188

23. Gray, 'Stimulus-dependent neuronal oscillations and local synchronisation in striate cortex of the alert', Cat Journal of Neuroscience 1 May 1997, 17(9) 3239-3253. Gamma Rhythm – an overview, Science direct.com

24. Davidson and Lutz, 'Buddhas brain: neuroplasticity and meditation', IEEE Signal Process Mag, 2008, Jan 1;25(1):176-174

25. Buszaki G, Rhythms of the brain, 2006,OUP. Nyhus E, Curran T, 'Functional role of gamma and theta oscillations in episodic memory', Neuroscience and Biobehavioral Reviews, June 2010, 34 (7): 1023-1035.

26. Laccarino et al, 'Gamma Frequency entrainment attenuates amyloid load and modifies microglia', Nature 540, 230-235, 8 December 2016

27. Lim et al, 'Photobiomodulation in the brain: a novel approach to treating Alzheimer's disease', Therapy in Neurology and Neuroscience 2019 pp.401–417

28. Ardeshirylajimi et al, 'Comprehensive overview on utilizing electromagnetic fields in bone regenerative medicine', Electromagnetic

Biology and Medicine Vol 38, 2019 – Issue 1

29. De Girolamo et al, 'Low frequency pulsed electromagnetic field affects proliferation, tissue-specific gene expression, and cytokines release of human tendon cells', Cell Biochem Biophys, 2013, Jul;66(3):697-708

30. Hannah Iaccarino et al, 'Gamma frequency entrainment attenuates amyloid load and modifies microglia', Nature, 8 Dec 2016;540,230-235

31. Amy Serin et al, 'The therapeutic effect of bilateral alternating stimulation tactile form technology on the stress response' Journal of Biotechnology and Biomedical Science. Issn No:2576-6694

32. Stagg CJ et al 'Physiological basis of transcranial Direct Current Stimulation'. The Neuroscientist Feb 22 2011, 17(1):37-53

33. Danilov YP and Kublanov VS, 'Emerging noninvasive neurostimulation technologies: CN, NINM and sympathy correction' Journal of Behavioral and Brain Science, 4, 2014, 105-113

34. Cichon N, Bijak M, Czarny P, Miller E, et al, ' Increase in blood levels of growth factors involved in the neuroplasticity process by using an extremely low frequency electromagnetic field in post-stroke patients', Front Aging Neurosci. 2018 Sep 26;10:294

35. As footnote 34 above

REFERENCE SECTION
Mind mechanics and brain specialists

1. Frederick Crews, 'Freud: the making of an illusion', 2017 New York: Metropolitan Books, Henry Holy & Company

Neurotransmitters and other chemical messengers – the fundamentals of brain function

1. www.quora.com/How-many-types-of-neurotransmitters-are-there-in-a-human-brain

2. Komiya M et al, 'Lemon oil vapor causes an anti stress effect via moulatig the 5-HTP and DA activities in mice', Behav Brain Res 2006 Sep 25;172(2):240-9

3. Kukkonen-Harjula K et al, 'Haemodynamic and hormonal responses to heat exposure in a Finnish sauna bath', Eur J AQppl Physiol Occup Physiol 1989;58(5):543-50

4. Kamal, Summary of Melatonin, Examine.com Sept 30 2018

5. Kristin Szuhany et al 'A meta-analytic review of the effects of exercise on brain-derived neurotrophic factor', Journal of Psychiatric research, 2015 Jan: 60:56-64

6. Reyes-Izquierdo et al, 'Modulatory effect of coffee fruit extract on plasma levels of brain-derived neurotropic factor in healthy subjects', Br J Nutr 2013 Aug28;110(3):420-5

7. Wattanathorn J et al, 'Positive modulation of cognition and mod in the health elderly volunteer following the administration of centella asiatica', J Ethnopharmacol, 5 Mar 2008;116(2):325-32

8. Juliana Phillips et al, 'Student's discovery draws interest from International scientific community', April 13, 2017, Greenville University, Illinois, USA

Brain-boosting psychobiotics

1. Timothy G Dinan and John F Cryan, 'Mood by microbe: towards clinical translation', 6 April 2016. Genome Medicine2016;8:36

2. Behav Brain Res. 2016 Feb 1;298(Pt B):202-9.

3. S Liang et al, 'Administration of Lactobacillus helveticus NS8 improves behavioural, cognitive, and biochemical aberrations caused by chronic restraint stress', Neuroscience. 2015 Dec 3;310:561-77

4. A Kato-Kataoka et al, 'Fermented milk containing Lactobacillus casei strain Shirota prevents the onset of physical symptoms in medical students under academic examination stress', Benef Microbes. 2016;7(2):153-6.O)

5. H M Savignac et al, 'Bifidobacteria modulate cognitive processes in an anxious mouse strain', Behavioural Brain Research vol 287 1 July 2015, pp.59-72

6. K Schmidt et al, 'Prebiotic intake reduces the waking cortisol response and alters emotional bias in healthy volunteers', Psychpharmacology, May 2015, Vol 232, Issue 10, pp 1793-1801

7. A Burokas et al, 'Targeting the microbiota-gut-brain axis: prebiotics have anxiolytic and antidepressant-like effects and reverse the impact of chronic stress in mice', Biological Psychiatry, Vol 82, Issue 7, 1 Oct 2017, pp.472-487

8. Christopher Lowry et al, 'Identification of an immune-responsive mesolimbocortical serotonergic system: potential role in regulation of emotional behavior', published online on March 28 in Neuroscience

9. Valles-Colomer et al, 'The neuroactive potential of the human gut microbiota in quality of life and depression', Nature Microbiology, 4 February 2019

Cannabis brain benefits

1. S Rieder et al, Cannabinoid-induced apoptosis in immune cells as a pathway to immunosuppression', Immunobiology, 2010 August, 215(8): 598-605.

INDEX

ACKNOWLEDGEMENTS

The author would like to thank the following for the images: p.19 Alexander Pokusay, 123FR.com, p.111 and p.204 Maa Illustrations; and to the American Institute for Stress for the use of the Holmes Rahe Stress scale calculator.

NOTES

NOTES

If you have enjoyed *Reboot Your Brain*, why not add Sara Davenport's *Reboot Your Health* to your library of health favourites?

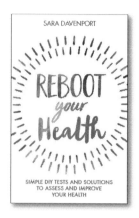

And if you would like to read in-depth articles on many of the topics in this book, please sign up for the fortnightly newsletter on www.reboothealth.co.uk and receive a free e-copy of my book *Understanding Alzheimer's* which retails at £6.99.

Reboot Your Health looks at all aspects of holistic health and healing, bringing you a regular dose of DIY get-well advice. From nutrition to detox, sleep to air pollution and the best health tests on the market, the blog covers a wide range of topics, delivering you the low-down on conventional medicine and complementary therapies. Check out the range of top tips, recipes and ideas on how to live better; sign up today for information on a whole host of brain relevant topics and find out about health experts who might just change your life. All free of charge and backed by science.

All your questions answered on topics such as:

Air pollution, Brain Fog, Pesticides, Lyme disease, Sleep, Mould, Detox, Candida, Electromagnetic fields and the arrival of 5G, Trigeminal Neuralgia, Brain biotics, Dementia, Toxic teeth, HIIT and exercise, Stem cells, Mental health apps

And many, many more.

Reboot Your Health – if you don't take care of yourself, who else is going to?

Printed in Great Britain
by Amazon

74530410R00179